Evidence-Based Trauma Pearls

Editors

JEANETTE VAUGHAN
WHITNEY VILLEGAS

CRITICAL CARE NURSING CLINICS OF NORTH AMERICA

www.ccnursing.theclinics.com

Consulting Editor
DEBORAH GARBEE

June 2023 • Volume 35 • Number 2

ELSEVIER

1600 John F. Kennedy Boulevard • Suite 1800 • Philadelphia, Pennsylvania, 19103-2899

http://www.theclinics.com

CRITICAL CARE NURSING CLINICS OF NORTH AMERICA Volume 35, Number 2
June 2023 ISSN 0899-5885, ISBN-13: 978-0-323-93933-1

Editor: Kerry Holland
Developmental Editor: Ann Gielou M. Posedio

Critical Care Nursing Clinics of North America (ISSN 0899-5885) is published quarterly by Elsevier Inc., 360 Park Avenue South, New York, NY 10010-1710. Months of issue are March, June, September, and December. Business and Editorial Offices: 1600 John F. Kennedy Blvd., Suite 1800, Philadelphia, PA 19103-2899. Periodicals postage paid at New York, NY and additional mailing offices. Subscription prices are $160.00 per year for US individuals, $456.00 per year for US institutions, $100.00 per year for US students and residents, $206.00 per year for Canadian individuals, $573.00 per year for Canadian institutions, $230.00 per year for international individuals, $573.00 per year for international institutions, $115.00 per year for international students/residents and $100.00 per year for Canadian students/residents. To receive student/resident rate, orders must be accompanied by name of affiliated institution, data of term, and the *signature* of program/residency coordinator on institution letterhead. Orders will be billed at individual rate until proof of status is received. Foreign air speed delivery is included in all *Clinics* subscription prices. All prices are subject to change without notice. **POSTMASTER:** Send address changes to *Critical Care Nursing Clinics of North America*, Elsevier Health Sciences Division, Subscription Customer Service, 3251 Riverport Lane, Maryland Heights, MO 63043. **Customer Service: 1-800-654-2452 (US and Canada); 314-447-8871 (outside US and Canada). Fax: 314-447-8029. E-mail:** JournalsCustomerService-usa@elsevier.com **(for print support) and** JournalsOnlineSupport-usa@elsevier.com **(for online support).**

Reprints. For copies of 100 or more of articles in this publication, please contact the Commercial Reprints Department, Elsevier Inc., 360 Park Avenue South, New York, New York, 10010-1710; Tel.: 212-633-3874, Fax: 212-633-3820, and E-mail: reprints@elsevier.com.

Critical Care Nursing Clinics of North America is covered in *MEDLINE/PubMed (Index Medicus), International Nursing Index, Nursing Citation Index, Cumulative Index to Nursing and Allied Health Literature, and RNdex Top 100.*

Contributors

CONSULTING EDITOR

DEBORAH GARBEE, PhD, APRN, ACNS-BC, FCNS
Associate Dean for Professional Practice, Community Service and Advanced Nursing Practice, Professor of Clinical Nursing, Louisiana State University Health Sciences Center New Orleans School of Nursing, New Orleans, Louisiana, USA

EDITORS

JEANETTE VAUGHAN, DNP, RN, CCRN, CNL
Instructor, Department of Nursing, Faculty Member, Texas A and M University, Commerce School of Nursing, Austin, Texas, USA

WHITNEY VILLEGAS, DNP, APRN, AGACNP-BC
Adjunct Nursing Faculty, Texas Tech University Health Sciences Center, Lubbock, Texas, USA; Geriatric Nurse Practitioner, Trauma Service, Advance Practice Provider, Trauma and Acute Care Surgery, JPS Health Network, Fort Worth, Texas, USA

AUTHORS

LORI AARON-BRIJA, DNP, APRN, FNP-C
Assistant Clinical Professor, Texas Woman's University, Dallas, Texas, USA

COLETTE BAUDOIN, PhD (c), MSN, RN, CNE, OCN
Instructor of Clinical Nursing, School of Nursing, Louisiana State University Health Sciences Center New Orleans, New Orleans, Louisiana, USA

EMILY BERKOWITZ, PhD, APRN, ANP-C, CVNP-BC, CNE
Assistant Professor, Texas Woman's University, Dallas, Texas, USA

HALLI CARR, DNP, APRN, ACNP-BC
Baylor Louise Herrington School of Nursing, Dallas, Texas, USA

DAMON B. COTTRELL, PhD, DNP, APRN, FNP-C, CCNS, ACNS-BC
Professor and Interim Dean, Texas Woman's University, Denton, Texas, USA; Nurse Practitioner, Village Medical, Little Elm, Texas, USA

ALISON H. DAVIS, PhD, RN, CNE, CHSE
Associate Professor of Clinical Nursing, School of Nursing, Louisiana State University Health Sciences Center New Orleans, New Orleans, Louisiana, USA

LIV DINOSO, DNP, PMHNP-BC, FNP-C, CNE
Instructor of Clinical Nursing, School of Nursing, Louisiana State University Health Sciences Center New Orleans, New Orleans, Louisiana, USA

ELEANOR R. FITZPATRICK, DNP, RN, AGCNS-BC, ACNP-BC, CCRN, CCCTM
Clinical Nurse Specialist, Surgical Intensive Care Unit, Thomas Jefferson University Hospital, Philadelphia, Pennsylvania, USA

SHANNON S. GAASCH, MS, CRNP, AGACNP-BC
University of Maryland Medical Center, R Adams Cowley Shock Trauma Center, Baltimore, Maryland, USA

ALEXANDRA HUNT, MSN, CRNP, AGACNP-BC
R Adams Cowley Shock Trauma Center, University of Maryland Medical Center, Baltimore, Maryland, USA

RENEE' JONES, DNP, APRN, WHNP-BC
Baylor Louise Herrington School of Nursing, Dallas, Texas, USA

CHRISTOPHER L. KOLOKYTHAS, MS, AGACNP-BC, ACCNS-AG, CRNP, APRN-CNS
University of Maryland Medical Center, R Adams Cowley Shock Trauma Center, Baltimore, Maryland, USA

QUINN LACEY, PhD, RN, CCRN
Nursing Instructor, School of Nursing, LSU Health-New Orleans, New Orleans, Louisiana, USA

TRACEY LAWSON, MSN, RN, CEN
Emergency Nurse Manager, Singleton District Hospital, New South Wales, Australia

AIMME J. McCAULEY, DNP, MSN, RN, CNE
Instructor of Clinical Nursing, School of Nursing, Louisiana State University Health Sciences Center New Orleans, New Orleans, Louisiana, USA

MAUREEN FRANCES McLAUGHLIN, MS, RN, ACNS-BC, CPAN, CAPA
Quality Nurse, Department of Anesthesiology, Lahey Hospital and Medical Center, Burlington, Massachusetts, USA

KAREN A. MCQUILLAN, MS, RN, CNS-BC, CCRN, CNRN, TCRN, FAAN
R Adams Cowley Shock Trauma Center, University of Maryland Medical Center, Baltimore, Maryland, USA

MARY RITTER, DNP, MSN, MLS, APRN, FNPBC
Assistant Professor, Southeastern Louisiana University, Hammond, Louisiana, USA; Advanced Practice Provider, Urgent Care, Premier Health, Baton Rouge, Louisiana, USA

JEANETTE VAUGHAN, DNP, RN, CCRN, CNL
Instructor, Department of Nursing, Faculty Member, Texas A and M University, Commerce School of Nursing, Austin, Texas, USA

WHITNEY VILLEGAS, DNP, APRN, AGACNP-BC
Adjunct Nursing Faculty, Texas Tech University Health Sciences Center, Lubbock, Texas, USA; Geriatric Nurse Practitioner, Trauma Service, Advance Practice Provider, Trauma and Acute Care Surgery, JPS Health Network, Fort Worth, Texas, USA

JJEFFREY WILLIAMS, DNP, APRN, CCNS
Associate Clinical Professor, Texas Woman's University, Dallas, Texas, USA

Contents

Trauma remains a leading cause of death among adults. Care of the trauma patient requires highly skilled trauma teams. Trauma care begins in the field, then presents to the emergency room, proceeds to intensive care in many cases, and finally reaches recovery and rehabilitation. For patients, it can be a long road. To be effective, multidisciplinary trauma teams must expertly drill and practice skills, communicate among team members in closed loops, make split decisions affecting patient outcomes, and see the care through to the end. Many disruptions during the course of providing trauma care can alter safe outcomes for patients. The American Association of Critical Care Nurses Six Essentials of the Healthy Work Environment are presented as a framework to provide excellence in trauma care, both for the patient and team members. The six essentials of a healthy work environment include skilled communication, true collaboration, effective decision-making, appropriate staffing, meaningful recognition, and authentic leadership.

Airway assessment and management is the first priority in trauma care. The airway can be compromised by traumatic injuries or altered mentation. Airway assessment is conducted during the primary survey. Airway triage in trauma is determined by patient and environmental factors. Initial interventions include positioning maneuvers and suction to clear the airway with supplemental oxygen. Endotracheal intubation and surgical (or "front of neck") airways are considered definitive. Traumatic airway injuries are rare but have high mortality and morbidity if undetected.

Traumatic cervical spinal cord injury can cause significant neurologic disability. A cervical spine injury impacts not only the neurologic system but also numerous other organ systems of the body. This complex injury requires a systematic approach to assessment and care aimed at preventing, recognizing, and treating potentially devastating secondary spinal cord injury and multisystem complications. This article focuses on the pathophysiology, initial presentation, and treatment of cervical spinal cord injury by body system.

The challenge in caring for patients who sustain traumatic chest injuries centers on their complex needs from high acuity and the potential for multisystem effects and complications. Hemorrhage and respiratory compromise are common sequela of thoracic trauma. Patients must be resuscitated and their injuries managed with the primary goals of restoring cardiopulmonary structural integrity and preventing complications. There are evolving strategies for the management of the thoracic trauma victim including damage control resuscitation and surgery, endovascular repairs, and assessments implementing severity scores to aid in planning interventions.

A patient with trauma presents a unique and/or complex challenge to the ethical foundation that guides nursing care. Patients with trauma, by the very nature of the suddenness of their injury, are unable to predetermine or express their wishes in the event of a catastrophic injury. The providers who care for patients with trauma do not have an established patient relationship to aid them in decision-making based on what they think the patient would wish or based on past conversations. Yet, they provide expert care and use ethical principles to direct their professional responsibility to these patients.

Geriatric trauma is increasing in the United States. The care of patients with geriatric trauma is complex due to age-related changes and comorbidities. Patients with geriatric trauma have increased risk of poor outcomes compared with younger patients with trauma, and the highest risk groups are those who have frailty. These patients require special care considerations. Multidisciplinary care can improve outcomes in frail patients with geriatric trauma.

Falls in the ICU are multifaceted, affecting patients of all ages. Historically, falls have been associated with patients in the hospital environment, but fall rates after discharge and readmission rates following a fall are now areas of concern. Recent innovations to prevent risks related to sedation and immobility in the hospital have revealed their impact on ICU patients and fall risk. Risk factors for falls in the ICU relate to length of stay and acuity-related care requirements, such as mechanical ventilation, sedation, and prolonged immobilization. Evidence-based fall prevention includes screening tools, prevention bundles/programs, and implementing clinical practice guidelines.

> Traumatic brain injury (TBI) is a leading cause of death and disability in the United States, predominantly impacting men. The highest risk for the development of a TBI includes athletes, construction workers, military personnel, and law enforcement. TBI is classified as mild, moderate, or severe. The degree of TBI will determine the severity of clinical manifestations. Management of TBI may be a combination of operative and non-operative interventions. Nursing considerations and management include frequent assessment of vital signs and neurologic status, maintaining hemodynamic stability, early identification of worsening clinical manifestations, and psychosocial support to the TBI patient and family.

> Trauma care is complex. Acute and critical care clinicians perceive trauma as a skilled response to critical injury or accident that occurs to patients, but trauma exists on many levels. One of those is a grim reality for patients who are lesbian, gay, bisexual, transgender, queer or questioning, and from other sexual and gender minorities (LGBTQ+). A lifetime of trauma through stigma, discrimination, and victimization is too often present. Owing to distrust of the health care system and clinicians, LGBTQ+ experience health and health care disparities.

> Traumatic injuries occur from unintentional and intentional violent events, claiming an estimated 4.4 million lives annually (World Health Organization). Abdominal trauma is a common condition seen in many trauma centers accounting for roughly 15% of all trauma-related hospitalizations (Boutros and colleagues 35) and is associated with significant morbidity and mortality. Following the concepts of Damage Control Resuscitation can reduce mortality drastically. Ultrasound, computed tomography scans, and routine physical examinations are used to make prompt diagnoses, trend injuries, and recognize deterioration of clinical status. Clear, effective, and closed-loop communication is essential to provide quality care.

> The authors provide a concise, comprehensive overview of the unique anatomic and physiologic features of pregnancy as well as modification and considerations important for the management of the pregnant trauma patient.

> Social determinants of health (SDOHs) have been well studied within the literature in the United States but the effects of these determinants of health on patients with trauma have garnered less attention. The interaction between patients with SDOHs and patients with trauma requires clinicians caring for this population to view patients with trauma through a multifaceted lens. The purpose of this article will be to illuminate the drivers of trauma in the adult population and how the SDOHs and the health-care system come together to contribute to disparities in trauma outcomes.

> Traumatic events such as hospitalization of family members in the intensive care setting can influence communication interactions between health-care workers and family members not just because of the acute situation but because it brings feelings resulting from past traumatic events to the surface. Providing trauma-informed care to all patients and families in the critical care setting improves communication and results in encounters that are less likely to result in an escalation of negative emotions and outbursts and provides an environment that is conducive to interprofessional communication between families, patients, and health-care workers.

CRITICAL CARE NURSING CLINICS OF NORTH AMERICA

SERIES OF RELATED INTEREST

Nursing Clinics of North America http://www.nursing.theclinics.com

THE CLINICS ARE AVAILABLE ONLINE!
Access your subscription at:
www.theclinics.com

Preface

Why Trauma Involves Many Issues

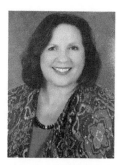
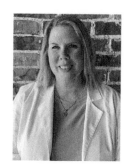

Jeanette Vaughan, DNP, RN, CCRN, CNL   Whitney Villegas, DNP, APRN, AGACNP-BC
Editors

Presentations of trauma experienced by patients today are far more complex than seen in previous decades. Patients are impacted by catastrophic pandemics, a brutal economy, and health care teams experiencing critical states of vacancy and battle fatigue. All of these factors affect safety and patient outcomes. Providing expert trauma care from both a physical and mental health standpoint is essential to manage complex cases. A diverse, expert, multidisciplinary team is a fundamental component not only to trauma resuscitation, but towards recovery. This issue begins with the essentials of a healthy work environment and how to establish a dynamic, well-trained, multidisciplinary trauma team. Also provided are several articles highlighting how mental health, LGBTQ+ matters, and social determinants of health impact trauma outcomes. Rounding out the issue are articles exploring current trends in trauma obstetrics, geriatric frailty, and cutting-edge strategies to manage polytrauma. Holistic trauma care includes repairing and recovering the body, mind, and spirit. Trauma is often fraught with ethical dilemmas. Trauma-informed care is key in providing pathways toward recovery. But most importantly of all, the reader will realize that expert trauma care is all about the team. From the first responders, to the ER, to the OR, and on to the ICU, a successful multidisciplinary trauma team begins with a healthy work environment. Each member of the team must embrace their role to work collaboratively in delivering evidence-based care. As practicing critical care nurses and educators, we hope that you find meaning in the articles presented in this issue which examine management of the complexities within trauma today.

Jeanette Vaughan, DNP, RN, CCRN, CNL
Texas A&M University Commerce School of Nursing
Greenville, TX, USA

Whitney Villegas, DNP, APRN, AGACNP-BC
Trauma Service
JPS Health
Fort Worth, TX, USA

E-mail addresses:
jeanette.vaughan@tamuc.edu (J. Vaughan)
Wvillega@jpshealth.org (W. Villegas)

Evidence-Based Pearls
How the Healthy Work Environment Effects Multidisciplinary Trauma Teams

Jeanette Vaughan, DNP, RN, CCRN, CNL

KEYWORDS

- Multidisciplinary trauma teams • Trauma-informed care
- Essentials healthy work envirnoment

KEY POINTS

- Ensuring healthy work environments benefit trauma teams.
- Effective trauma teams include componets of trauma informed care.
- Expert multdisciplinary trauma teams not only follow traditional A,B,C,D primary surveys, but explore complex emotional and mental health issues.

Trauma. It is gritty. It is gory. To some, it is an adrenalin fix. Trauma can be an act of violence or purely an accident. Trauma continues to be the leading cause of death among people from 1 to 46 in the United States.[1] Trauma is almost always unexpected for the victim, and stress for the victims and their families is inherent. Those who have worked in trauma emergency departments, served trauma patients in the field, or managed survivors in intensive care units (ICUs) know these facts. Trauma victims survive through the careful and timely management of care delivered by expert, multidisciplinary trauma teams. Essential to that team is a healthy work environment.

In August 2022, the American Association of Critical Care Nurses (AACN) released The National Nurse Work Environments–October 2021: Status Report. Their findings point out that overall the health of nurses' work environments have suffered a dramatic decline, even since 2018.[2] Reasons for the decline include age-old systemic problems, such as staffing and moral distress. Current data indicate that those issues have reached a breaking point, with more than 67% of critical care nurses planning to leave their current positions within the next 3 years.[3] In addition, 72% reported having suffered at least one violent or harmful work event involving verbal abuse, physical abuse, discrimination, or sexual harassment.[2] Now, more than ever, to foster optimal patient outcomes, health-care teams must strive to address the standards of a healthy work environment.[3] A healthy work environment includes skilled communication, true collaboration, effective decision-making, authentic leadership, meaningful recognition,

Texas A and M University Commerce, Department of Nursing, 2210 Highway 24, Commerce, TX 75429, USA
E-mail address: jeanette.vaughan@tamuc.edu

Crit Care Nurs Clin N Am 35 (2023) 101–107
https://doi.org/10.1016/j.cnc.2023.02.002
0899-5885/23/© 2023 Elsevier Inc. All rights reserved.

skilled communication, and appropriate staffing.[4] Healthy work environments empower team members to provide quality care and provide healing for both staff and patients.[5] Because nursing is inherently linked to improved patient outcomes, healthy, emotionally balanced, and supported team members are essential to that work.[2,5]

SKILLS OF THE TRAUMA TEAM

Effective communication by expert team members is essential to successfully resuscitate the trauma patient for positive outcomes. In their 2020 guidelines, the American Heart Association stresses the gold-standard importance of closed-loop communication and teamwork to enhance survival when providing advanced life support.[6] The Joint Commission identified poor communication as a root cause of sentinel events.[7] Conversely, a meta-analysis by Lake and associates showed that healthy work environments are linked to lower numbers of safety incidents, mortality, and poor patient outcomes.[8]

To effectively resuscitate patients, the trauma team must be skilled in situational awareness.[9] Situational awareness assists critical decision-making during intense, quickly changing crises during trauma resuscitation.[10] Checklists and visual prompts in the resuscitation bay can enhance and direct time-critical interventions.[11] Multidisciplinary trauma teams can be trained in situational awareness through the Team Situation Awareness Global Assessment Technique, a valid and reliable simulation-based method.[10] Although simulation has been shown to improve the performance of multidisciplinary team, additional behavior change techniques are required to advance intervention from the training environment to actual practice.[11] In China, a group of trauma surgeons realized that fragmentation of care occurred when the patient left the emergency department. Zhong and colleagues[12] piloted a temporary-sustainable follow-through team of consultants and found significant advantages in the model over the traditional multidisciplinary team model when providing care for severely injured trauma patients.

TRAUMA ROLES

The multidisciplinary team plays a vital role in trauma outcomes. Trauma teams in the emergency room typically consist of an attending trauma surgeon, senior residents, an orthopedic surgeon, a neurosurgeon on-call, the primary trauma nurse, a secondary trauma nurse, a respiratory therapist, medics, a radiology technician, and a chaplain. The trauma patient advocate is a newer role within the team to assist patients and families in understanding the complexities of trauma and navigating the road to long-term recovery.[13] Another key role is that of the receiving ICU team. Many have heard the phrase, "There is no 'I' in team." To successfully resuscitate, the trauma patient requires expert trauma team members who communicate to share findings that ensure positive patient outcomes.

The multidisciplinary team approach must continue when the patient is transferred to the ICU. Many units utilize grand rounds to ensure the completion of this task. Communication and continuity between emergency trauma teams, the trauma coordinators, and care providers of the ICUs are essential for ongoing successful inpatient treatment.[12] Establishing a trauma team leader to follow-up and manage the trauma patient in the ICU has been suggested as beneficial for the overall outcomes of trauma patients.[1] The trauma team leader helps to coordinate the roles required within the multidisciplinary team. Learning the nontechnical skills of team composition, roles, responsibilities, procedural compliance, and leadership can enhance real-world trauma resuscitation.[9] The coronavirus disease 2019 pandemic substantiated the ongoing need for outstanding trauma team dynamics, making the continuing training and resilience of trauma teams vital to improved resuscitation outcomes.[14]

THE IMPORTANCE OF HEALTHY WORK ENVIRONMENTS

As essential members of the multidisciplinary trauma team, nurses need to focus on psychological health and well-being to reduce burnout, job dissatisfaction, and intent to leave the critical care environment.[15,16] Teams and units must be adequately staffed to provide optimal trauma patient outcomes. When teams experience poor working environments with poor communication, errors and ineffective care delivery occur, contributing to conflicts among providers.[17] An unhealthy climate within a team directly translates to care being delivered.[18]

Communication among teams is threaded throughout the research on effective trauma resuscitation teams. It also appears in several facets of AACN's 6 essentials of a healthy work environment (**Fig. 1**). A healthy work environment encompasses

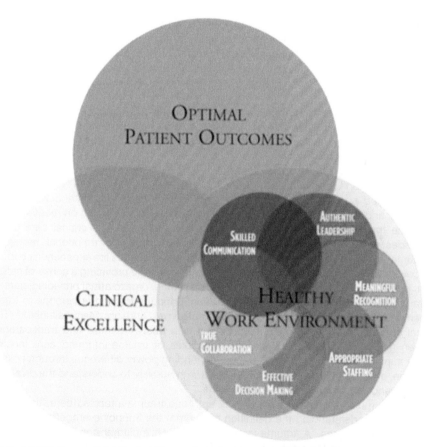

Fig. 1. AACN's 6 essentials of a healthy work environment. American Association of Critical-Care Nurses. AACN Standards for Establishing and Sustaining Healthy Work Environments: A Journey to Excellence. 2nd ed. Aliso Viejo, CA: AACN; 2016. https://www.aacn.org/WD/HWE/Docs/HWEStandards.pdf. ©2016 by the American Association of Critical-Care Nurses. All rights reserved. Used with permission.

safety, empowering the team, and satisfying participants.[16] Team communication and recognition enhance the camaraderie and satisfaction key to a work environment.[19]

Another factor affecting teams is bullying. Bullying can include microaggression, lateral violence, and horizontal hostility.[20] American Association of Critical Care Nurses (AACN) asserts bullying can contribute to nurse burnout, turnover, and poor patient outcomes.[2] The bullying phenomenon is documented throughout team literature and spans from nursing school students to executive leadership.[20] Bullying in critical care not only increases health-care costs due to turnover but also potentiates safety risks to patients.[2] A significant percentage of nurses leave their first job due to bullying, which simply has no place among highly functional teams.[20] See **Fig. 1** for an example of the 6 essentials of a healthy work environment and its overarching themes.

SAFETY OF TRAUMA-INFORMED CARE

The American Nurses Association created the Nurses' Bill of Rights to highlight best practices within health-care environments that benefit nurses and patient outcomes.[21] Included in those rights are providing a safe working environment for themselves and patients and a workplace that supports ethical practice and professional standards.[22] The 2030 Future of Nursing Report's mission is for nurses to chart a path toward health equity as set forth by the National Academies of Science, Engineering, and Medicine (NASEM).[23] By ensuring providers work in a healthy environment, the goal of providing equitably, quality health care to all persons is achieved. Within the report, NASEM emphasizes that nurses are often the first person with whom a patient encounter occurs. As the most trusted professionals on the team, nurses are integral in helping patients and themselves live their healthiest lives. As such, NASEM has set the standard that to accomplish health equity, nurses need robust education, supportive work environments, and autonomy.[23]

Another key ingredient of a successful trauma team is providing trauma-informed care. The Robert Wood Johnson Foundation and the Center for Health Care Strategies have funded research to advance trauma-informed care. Understanding that the physical and emotional effects of trauma have long-lasting impacts on recovery.[24,25] For the trauma patient, resuscitation is just the first step. The critical care nurse provides the ongoing tenets of a complete physical and emotional recovery. Trauma-informed care includes understanding how a patient's life experiences impact recovery. Core principles of trauma-informed care include providing a sense of safety for patients, their families, the staff, and the entire organization providing care.[26] Trauma-informed care should enhance patient engagement and adherence to treatment regimes, thus promoting improved outcomes and provider wellness.[24] The goal of building trust in trauma care begins with trustworthiness and transparency when making decisions.[26] Other core principles of trauma-informed care include peer support among team members, understanding power difference through collaboration, empowerment, and responsiveness with humility to understand the diversity, equity, and inclusion of all types of patients.

For the multidisciplinary team to fully embrace trauma-informed care, they must begin with understanding the definition of trauma; the 3 Es of event, effect, and the patient's experience. A trauma-informed approach includes comprehending how the trauma affects the patient via the 4 Rs: realization, recognition, response, and resistance to retraumatization.[27] A well-trained, successful, healthy trauma team utilizes various methods of knowing. Zander explored attributes of the ways of knowing and found resemblance to the sentinel work of Carper (1978), who suggested that ways of knowing include an empirical foundation of thinking, a moral component of

Table 1	
Comparison of healthy work environments and trauma-informed approaches	
AACN's Six Essentials of a Healthy Work Environment	**Trauma-Informed Approaches**
Skilled communication	Clear communications
True collaboration	Training and support of all staff
Authentic leadership	Steady leadership
Effective decision-making	Organizational policy development on trauma-informed care
Meaningful recognition	Engagement of patients in planning
Appropriate staffing	Higher and training of trauma-informed workforces

Note: Information sourced from *AACN's Six Essentials of a Healthy Work Environment* and a white paper on *Key Ingredients for Successful Trauma-Informed Care Implementation.*

ethics, esthetics or the art of nursing, and personal knowing, which means an understanding of self and others.[28] As one can see, many of the tenants of trauma-informed care resemble the essentials of a healthy work environment. Commonalities include clear communication, steady leadership, and the creation of safe emotional and physical work environments. The engagement of patients is also critical in the development process, similar to trauma grand rounds and ongoing training to provide a trauma-informed workforce. See **Table 1** for a side-by-side comparison of the 6 essentials of a healthy work environment and trauma-informed care approaches.

SUMMARY

The goal of the Precision Medicine Initiative launched by President Barack Obama in 2015 is to deliver "the right treatments, at the right time, every time to the right person."[29] To advance this initiative, nurses play a vital role through their day-to-day assessment, health history taking, patient education, and monitoring.[30] By threading the essentials of a healthy work environment across multidisciplinary teams, the health-care provider can master techniques to best manage the complex trauma patients of today. Promoting and sustaining a healthy work environment is a continuous effort.[16] A patient's trauma outcomes are only as good as the overall vitality and professionalism of the multidisciplinary team. Teams must work toward equality and equal beneficence of all members in training to be truly effective.[31,32] The American Psychiatric Nurses Association asserts that whole health begins with mental health, not only of patients but also of providers, and includes body, mind, and spirit.[29] As a public health-care issue, providers must recognize how the life-long impacts of trauma affect not only a patient's physical health but also their emotional health and social outcomes.[24]

CLINICS CARE POINTS

- Trauma teams must recognize and value all multidisciplinary team members equally.
- Failure to ensure that trauma teams strive to provide health work envirnoments ultimately effects patient outcomes negatively.

REFERENCES

1. Lavigueur O, Nemeth J, Razek T, et al. The effect of a multidisciplinary trauma team leader paradigm at a tertiary trauma center: 10-year experience. Emergency Medicine International 2020;2020. 8412179-8.

2. Ulrich B., Cassidy L., Barden C., et al., National nurse work environments – October 2021: a status report, *Crit Care Nurse*, 42, 2022, 58-70.

3. Bettancourt A., AACN national work environments study results [letter].American Association of Critical Care Nurses, Available at: www.aacn.org. Accessed July 13, 2022, 2022.

4. Barden C. AACN standards for establishing and sustaining a healthy work environment: A journey to excellence. 2nd Ed. American Association of Critical Care Nurses; 2016.

5. Samoya A, Crutcher TD, Pilon BA. Maintaining healthy work environments. Nurs Crit Care 2015;10:1–7.

6. Magid DJ, Aziz K, Cheng A, et al. Part 2: evidence evaluation and guidelines development: 2020 american heart association guidelines for cardiopulmonary resuscitation and emergency cardiovascular care. Circulation 2020;142: S358–65.

7. The Joint Commission Center for Transforming Healthcare. Targeted solutions Tool® for hand-off communications. Oakbrook Terrace, Illinois: The Joint Commission; 2017.

8. Lake ET, Sanders J, Duan R, et al. A meta-analysis of the associations between the nurse work environment in hospitals and 4 sets of outcomes. Med Care 2019; 57(5):353–61.

9. Murphy M, Curtis K, McCloughen A. Facilitators and barriers to the clinical application of teamwork skills taught in multidisciplinary simulated Trauma Team Training. Injury 2019;50:1147–52.

10. Crozier MS, Ting HY, et al. Use of human patient simulation and validation of the team situation awareness global assessment technique (TSAGAT): a multidisciplinary team assessment tool in trauma education. J Surg Educ 2015;72: 156–63, 2014.

11. Murphy M, McCloughen A, Curtis K. Using theories of behaviour change to transition multidisciplinary trauma team training from the training environment to clinical practice. Implement Sci 2019;14:43.

12. Zhong X, Wen X, Ji C, et al. A temporary-sustainable team: a new multidisciplinary team model for severe trauma. Chin J Traumatol 2020;23:363–6.

13. Hartwell J, Albanese K, Retterer A, et al. A trauma patient advocate is a valuable addition to the multidisciplinary trauma team: a process improvement project. Am Surg 2016;82:183–5.

14. Johnson GGRJ, Beaumont J, Paton-Gay JD, et al. Multidisciplinary, multisite trauma team training during COVID-19: lessons from the first virtual E-S.T.A.R.T.T. course. Can J Surg 2021;64:609–E612.

15. Montgomery AP, Patrician PA, Azuero A. Nurse burnout syndrome and work environment impact patient safety grade. J Nurs Care Qual 2022;37(1):87–93.

16. Wei H, Sewell KA, Woody G, et al. The state of the science of nurse work environments in the United States: a systematic review. International Journal of Nursing Sciences 2018;5:287–300.

17. Blake N. The nurse leader's role in supporting healthy work environments. AACN Adv Crit Care 2015;26:201–3.

18. Li J, Talari P, Kelly A, et al. Interprofessional Teamwork Innovation Model (ITIM) to promote communication and patient-centered, coordinated care. BMJ Qual Saf 2018;27:700–70.
19. Connor JA, Ziniel SI, Porter C, et al. Interprofessional use and validation of the AACN healthy work environment assessment tool. Am J Crit Care 2018;27:363–71.
20. Edmonson C, Zelonka C. Our own worst enemies: the nurse bullying epidemic. Nurs Adm Q 2019;43:274–9.
21. Pryor LA. Know your rights. Nephrol Nurs J 2020;47:395–6.
22. Ulrich B. The transformation of nursing and health care the stars have aligned to unleash the power of nurses. Nephrol Nurs J 2021;48:223–98.
23. National Academies of Sciences, Engineering, and Medicine. The future of nursing 2020-2030: charting a path to achieve health equity. Washington, DC: The National Academies Press; 2021. https://doi.org/10.17226/25982.
24. Menschner C. and Maul, *Issue brief: Key ingredients for successful trauma-informed care implementation*, 2016, Center for Healthcare Strategies. Available at: https://www.samhsa.gov/sites/default/files/programs_campaigns/childrens_mental_health/atc-whitepaper-040616.pdf
25. Manian N, Rog DJ, Lieberman L, et al. The organizational trauma-informed practices tool (O-TIPs): development and preliminary validation. J Community Psychol 2022;50:515–40.
26. Substance abuse and mental health services administration. SAMHSA's concept of trauma and guidance for a trauma-informed approach. HHS publication No. (SMA administration, 2014. SAMHSA's concept of trauma and guidance for a trauma-informed approach. Rockville, MD: Substance Abuse and Mental Health Services, Available at: https://youth.gov/feature-article/samhsas-concept-trauma-and-guidance-trauma-informed-approach 14-4884. Accessed July 02, 2022.
27. Lathan EC, Selwyn CN, Langhinrichsen-Rohling J. The "3 Es" of trauma-informed care in a federally qualified health center: traumatic Event- and Experience-related predictors of physical and mental health Effects among female patients. J Community Psychol 2021;49(2):703–24.
28. Zander PE. Ways of knowing in nursing: the historical evolution of a concept. J Theor Construct Test 2007;11:7.
29. Obama BH. Remarks by the president on precision medicine. Office of the Press Secretary 2015 Jan 30. Available at: https://obamawhite hourse.archived.gov/the-press-office/2015/01/30/remarks-president-precision-medicine.
30. Lebet R, Joseph PV, Aroke EN. Knowledge of precision medicine and health care: an essential nursing competency. Am J Nurs 2019;119:34.
31. Gillman LM, Brindley P, Edin PG, et al. Simulated Trauma and Resuscitation Team Training course—evolution of a multidisciplinary trauma crisis resource management simulation course. Am J Surg 2016;212:188–93.e3, 2015.
32. American Psychiatric Nurses Association, Whole health begins with mental health, let it begin with you: self care tip sheet for nurses, Available at: https://www.apna.org/wp-content/uploads/2021/03/APNASelfCareTipSheet.pdf. Accessed July 01, 2022.

Airway Management in Trauma Patients

Whitney Villegas, DNP, APRN, AGACNP-BC[a,b,*], Tracey Lawson, MSN, RN, CEN[c,1]

KEYWORDS:

- Airway • Trauma • Injury

KEY POINTS

- Airway management is the first priority in trauma patients, and multiple factors can cause airway compromise.
- Airway interventions include repositioning, suction, utilization of airway adjuncts, and definitive airway placement.
- A definitive airway, a cuffed tube that is secured distal to the vocal cords, is generally indicated in patients with a Glascow Coma Score of 8 or less.
- Traumatic airway injuries are rare but have a high mortality and morbidity.

INTRODUCTION

The first priority in the care of the trauma patient is to establish a protected and unobstructed airway, because loss of airway causes rapid deterioration and death.[1,2] Various traumatic injuries can di'rectly compromise the airway, including upper and lower airway lacerations, facial burns and inhalation, and facial fractures. The airway can become obstructed by blood, debris, secretions, vomitus, edema, or dislodged teeth. Patients with altered consciousness from head injuries or intoxication may also have impaired airway protection.[1]

The upper airway includes the nasal passages, mouth, pharynx, and larynx above the vocal cords. The larynx below the vocal cords, trachea, bronchi, and bronchioles makeup the lower airway.[1,3] Compromise to any area of the airway risks inadequate ventilation, leading to hypoxia, tissue hypoxemia, morbidity, and mortality.[4] Within the guidelines of Advanced Trauma Life Support (ATLS), trauma care providers must be able to assess the airway, recognize the need for airway intervention, establish a patent airway, have alternative plans for failed airway attempts, assess for correct placement of artificial airways, and secure the airway to prevent displacement.[1]

[a] Texas Tech University, Lubbock, TX, USA; [b] JPS Health Network, 1500 South Main Street, Fort Worth, TX 76104, USA; [c] Singleton District Hospital, 25 Danger Street Singleton, New South Wales 2330, Australia
[1] Present address: 13 Valentine Close, Greta, New South Wales 2334, Australia.
* Corresponding author. 1500 South Main Street, Fort Worth, TX 76104.
E-mail addresses: Whitney.villegas@ttuhsc.edu; wvillega@jpshealth.org

Crit Care Nurs Clin N Am 35 (2023) 109–118
https://doi.org/10.1016/j.cnc.2023.02.003
0899-5885/23/© 2023 Elsevier Inc. All rights reserved.
ccnursing.theclinics.com

AIRWAY ASSESSMENT

The primary assessment of the trauma patient starts with the letter "A" for airway. If this assessment is being performed in the field or upon arrival to the emergency department, cervical spine precautions should also be maintained. The airway can be quickly assessed by asking the patient their name and what happened; the ability to speak clearly can easily rule out major airway compromise. Both the nasopharynx and oropharynx should also be inspected for foreign bodies, edema, lacerations, or other signs of obstruction. Potential airway compromise from facial trauma (ie, Lacerations, abrasions, or swelling) or mandible instability should be recognized.[1,5]

Physical examination findings for patients with airway obstruction and impending respiratory failure are outlined in **Box 1**. Respiratory distress, agitation, and noisy breathing can indicate airway obstruction or impending respiratory failure.[5] Patients who are considered abusive or belligerent may be hypoxic instead of intoxicated, and patients who refuse to lie flat may be struggling to maintain a patent airway.[1] Other factors to consider with airway protection include level of consciousness, the ability to cough clear secretions, and nausea or vomiting.[4]

AIRWAY TRIAGE

Trauma patients present multiple unique challenges affecting airway triage.[4] Airway management is individualized for each trauma patient through careful consideration of patient complexity, the urgency of the patient's situation, and environmental factors.[1,4] Some practicing nurses get confused regarding how important airway might be due to the American Heart Association (AHA)'s ongoing practice guidelines for resuscitation. Following a 5-year study in 2010, which found that compression-only cardiopulmonary resuscitation conducted by bystanders improved patient outcomes, the AHA switched its algorithms to C-A-B or cardiac-airway-breathing. This switch was based on coronary perfusion pressures. The AHA found and still maintains that rapid compressions of 100 beats a minute with limited interruptions improves the oxygenation to the brain by circulating what remaining oxygen is in the bloodstream.[6] Therefore, the practice for saving patients without a pulse is C-A-B. In all other

---

Box 1
Examination findings in airway compromise and impending respiratory failure

Signs of Airway Obstruction[1]
- Agitation
- Cyanosis (late finding)
- Retractions
- Use of accessory muscles
- Noisy breathing (stridor, gurgling)
- Dysphonia (hoarse voice)
- Inability to lie flat

Signs of Inadequate Ventilation[1]
- Asymmetric chest wall movement
- Decreased or absent breath sounds
- Tachypnea
- Labored breathing
- Poor oxygenation on blood gas
- Oxygen desaturation
- Hypoventilation on blood gas or continuous capnograph

resuscitation instances, where the patient does have a pulse, it is always about the airway. The airway continues to be important to the AHA, but research show that the patient outcomes when patients were pulseless were improved when time was not wasted by untrained caregivers struggling with airways.

Patient Factors

Multiple traumatic injuries necessitate the placement of a definitive airway, a tube inserted into the trachea below the vocal cords.[1] If there is any doubt of the patient's ability to maintain airway integrity, definitive airway placement should be performed.[1,7] A common threshold for intubation is a Glasgow Coma Score of 8 or lower. Patients with facial burns and potential inhalation injury, severe edema from other burns, and facial fractures with hemorrhage and edema may require a definitive airway to maintain patency. Patients with bilateral mandible body fractures may lose structural support to keep the airway open. Severe neck trauma can result in airway injury or hematoma that compresses or displaces the airway.[1]

Trauma patients with inadequate ventilation from traumatic injuries should also have a definitive airway placed for mechanical ventilation.[1] Pain from thoracic trauma (such as rib fractures) can result in rapid, shallow breathing, leading to eventual respiratory failure. Patients with head injuries may exhibit an abnormal, inadequate breathing pattern. Loss of respiratory muscle tone can result from injury, anesthesia, sedation, and muscle relaxers. High spinal cord injury can affect respiratory muscle control, necessitating artificial airway placement. Although spinal cord injuries below the third cervical spine preserve diaphragm function, control of the intercostal and abdominal muscles is lost, resulting in diaphragmatic or "abdominal" breathing.[1]

Pediatric, geriatric, and pregnant patients have anatomic and physiologic differences from adult trauma patients that require special considerations in monitoring and airway techniques (**Table 1**). Children have an abundance of physiologic reserve and may not exhibit signs of distress until respiratory failure occurs.[1] Conversely, geriatric patients and those with preexisting pulmonary dysfunction have reduced reserve and higher risk of respiratory failure after trauma. Pregnant patients have increased oxygen consumption and airway edema, increasing the risks of hypoxia with trauma and difficult intubation.[1,7] Each of these special populations should be closely monitored for subtle signs of impending respiratory failure.

Patients with a "difficult airway" are those who present challenges with endotracheal intubation, bag-valve-mask (BVM) ventilation, ventilation through a subglottic airway, or placing a surgical airway.[4] Patients who are prone to have difficult airways include those with a short muscular neck, receding chin, overbite, or limited mouth opening.[1,8] Patients with penetrating or blunt neck trauma can present difficulties with any type of airway.[4] BVM may be difficult in patients older than 50 years and those with history of obstructive sleep apnea, facial trauma, and facial hair.[4,7] The inability to extend the neck due to actual or suspect cervical spine injury or arthritis can also make intubation challenging.[1,4]

Environmental Factors

Trauma patients are frequently encountered by first responders in the field, where limited resources are available. Airway maintenance is a top priority in the prehospital setting, along with minimizing scene time. Artificial airways are often not necessary, allowing for faster transport to the trauma facility.[2] For patients who require artificial airway placement, prehospital intubation is technically difficult; rescue airways such as laryngeal mask airway or, rarely, cricothyroidotomy may be necessary.[2] In general, the emergency department is a more controlled environment with more resources for

Table 1
Airway Considerations in Special Populations

Population	Anatomic/Physiologic Variant	Consideration
Pediatric	• Short trachea[1] • Acute angle of nasopharynx toward the glottis[1] • Narrow airway at the cricoid ring[1]	• Monitor for tube displacement with any head movement[1] • Avoid nasotracheal intubation[1] • Uncuffed endotracheal tube for age <8[5]
Geriatric	• Presence of dentures may obstruct the airway[1] • Decreased medication metabolism[1] • Increased risk of respiratory failure[1] • Mouth and spine more rigid, enlarged tongue, decreased protective reflexes[1]	• Remove dentures if obstructing the airway; if no obstruction, leave in place during BVM to improve mask fit[1] • Reduce dosages of sedation and opioids[1] • Monitor closely for respiratory failure • Prepare for difficult airway
Pregnancy	• Increased oxygen consumption[6] • Hypocapnia common in late pregnancy[1] • Airway edema[6] • Decreased gastric emptying with aspiration risk[6]	• Monitor closely for respiratory failure with blood gas • Preoxygenation is critical prior to intubation[6] • Be prepared with adjunct for difficult airway[6]

airway management. If the patient arrives intubated, tube placement should be confirmed.[2] In all environments, team dynamics play a role in airway decision-making. It is important to consider the makeup of the team, as well as the skill set and level of experience of each member. For example, rural health care facilities may not have providers experienced in surgical airway.

Environmental considerations include the following:

- What care is needed? What resources are readily available?
- What skills can be performed by each team member?
- What is the initial airway plan? What is the next course of action if that plan fails?
- Are airway specialists (ie, anesthesia or ear-nose-throat) available if needed?

AIRWAY INTERVENTIONS AND ARTIFICIAL AIRWAYS

The initial interventions for a patient with a compromised airway are to optimize the patient's position and clear the airway.[1] Oral, nasal, and nasotracheal suction can help clear blood, debris, and secretions obstructing the airway. Patients with full stomachs and decreased level of consciousness are at high risk of vomiting and aspiration during airway interventions. If vomiting occurs in a patient with possible spinal injury, oral suction should be performed and the patient entirely rotated (by logroll) to a lateral position. The airway can also be opened with a chin-lift or jaw-thrust maneuver.[1,2,5]

Oropharyngeal and nasopharyngeal airways can be used temporarily to open the airway to allow for ventilation. In patients without airway reflexes (cough or gag), an oropharyngeal airway can be inserted behind the tongue to alleviate occlusion and facilitate BVM ventilation.[1,5] In adult patients, the oropharyngeal airway is inserted upside down with the curved portion directed upward toward the roof of the mouth; once contact is made with the soft palate, it is rotated 180° over the tongue.[1] However, the rotating technique should not be used in children due to increased risk of damage to the mouth and pharynx. Instead, a tongue blade is used to depress the tongue for insertion. A nasopharyngeal airway (also called "nasal trumpets") is inserted into the patient's nostril and advanced into the posterior oropharynx.[1] Nasal trumpets can be used on patients who are alert but is contraindicated in some patterns of facial fractures.[1,5]

To avoid hypoxia in trauma patients, supplemental oxygen can be administered by nasal cannula or mask. BVM ventilation is commonly used to assist ventilation in patients who are apneic, hypoxic, or have increased work of breathing to preoxygenate before definitive airway placement.[5] For successful BVM ventilation, the airway must remain patent with good seal of mask around the nose and mouth.[5] Dentures should be left in place during BVM to facilitate a good mask seal unless they cause airway obstruction.[6]

Extra-Glottic Airways

Extra-glottic airways are typically used in trauma patients temporarily as a bridge to obtaining a definitive airway. The laryngeal mask airway (LMA) is useful in emergency situations (before hospitalization or in the emergency department) to ventilate patients with difficult airways but is prone to inappropriate positioning.[1,2] The LMA can cause gastric insufflation and does not prevent aspiration.[2] Similar to the LMA, the laryngeal tube airway (LTA) can be placed without direct visualization.[1] The LMA and LTA are available in models that allow for endotracheal intubation through the device. A multi-lumen esophageal airway, or esophageal-tracheal device, is used mainly in trauma patients before hospitalization by first responders.[1] This device is blindly inserted into the oropharynx; one port terminates in the esophagus and is occluded with a balloon to allow ventilation through port within the trachea. Each extra-glottic airway should be verified by lung auscultation and end-tidal carbon dioxide monitoring.[5]

Endotracheal Tubes

The first-line definitive airway for patients with airway compromise or inadequate ventilation is endotracheal intubation, where a cuffed tube is inserted through the pharynx, past the vocal cords, and into the trachea. The most common method of intubation is the rapid sequence intubation (RSI), which uses the simultaneous administration of sedation and neuromuscular blocker with cricoid pressure to quickly insert an orotracheal tube.[4,5] The nasotracheal approach requires less sedation but is more time-consuming and inappropriate in patients with fractures of the frontal sinus, basilar skull, and cribriform plate.[1,5] Specific patient populations who can maintain respirations and are not in immediate danger of airway loss can undergo an awake intubation.[4] Awake intubation avoids sedation and uses topical medications for endotracheal tube insertion.[4]

After insertion, the cuff of the endotracheal tube must be inflated followed by BVM ventilation. Proper placement of the tube within the trachea is assessed by connecting an end-tidal carbon dioxide detector and observing for color change with BVM inhalation and exhalation. Auscultation of bilateral lung fields should illicit breath sounds without rumbling or gurgling in the epigastric area.[1] The tube is secured at a depth of approximately 21 cm in women or 23 cm in men from the corner of the mouth. A chest radiograph should be obtained to confirm proper depth.[2]

Video laryngoscopy can give clearer views of the glottis and provide higher success rates in patients with difficult airways, cervical immobilization, and by inexperienced providers.[2,8] Trauma providers can also elect to use an intubating LMA or LTA as bridge to definitive airway or a gum elastic bougie (GEB) to assist with intubation of an anatomically anterior airway.[1,2,8] When the vocal cords cannot be visualized, the provider can blindly pass the GEB into the epiglottis and then thread the endotracheal tube over it.[1]

Endotracheal intubation should be halted for significant desaturations to prevent complications.[9] If intubation fails, the trauma team reverts to basic airway management (jaw-trust and pharyngeal airway) with BVM ventilation.[1] The patient should be oxygenated back to 100% oxygen saturation, if possible, to give more time for the next attempt.[2] Hypoxic brain injury occurs at approximately 6 minutes of apnea, and more than 2 passes at intubation is associated with significant increases in aspiration, hypothermia, and cardiac arrest.[7,9] The Western Trauma Association guidelines suggest placement of a surgical airway after 3 intubation attempts or a time of 10 minutes without a definitive airway.[2]

SURGICAL AIRWAYS

Trauma patients with edema of the glottis, laryngeal fracture, airway obstruction from oropharyngeal or neck hemorrhage, or inability to place an endotracheal tube should undergo placement of a surgical airway to allow for ventilation and adequate oxygenation.[1] Surgical airways may also be called "front of neck airways". Cricothyroidotomy can be performed quickly in emergent situations by either the needle or the surgical approach. In needle cricothyroidotomy, a 12- or 14-gauge needle is inserted into the cricothyroid membrane, allowing for safe oxygenation for 30 to 45 minutes until intubation or formal tracheostomy can be performed. This technique is a temporary airway measure because it does not allow for adequate exhalation, resulting in carbon dioxide accumulation.[1] Surgical cricothyroidotomy is performed by making an incision in the cricothyroid membrane and inserting a small endotracheal or tracheostomy tube. This procedure should not be done in patients younger than 12 years.[1]

Tracheostomy tubes are not recommended by ATLS guidelines for emergent surgical airway placement, because they take more time than a cricothyroidotomy and can result in profuse bleeding.[1] Trauma patients commonly undergo tracheostomy placement in controlled situations to replace an emergent cricothyroidotomy or establish a long-term airway.[9] The faster percutaneous approach to tracheostomy has reduced infection rates, whereas the open technique is indicated in high-risk patients.[9]

TRAUMA NURSING ROLE IN AIRWAY MANAGEMENT

The nurse plays a critical role in trauma airway assessment, intervention, and maintenance. Depending on available resources and defined team roles, the nurse may be highly involved in definitive airway procedures (**Box 2**). Nursing duties during intubation include patient preparation, gathering equipment, administration of medications, and hemodynamic monitoring.[1,2,5] In preparing for intubation, every airway should be presumed difficult with a variety of airway adjuncts and difficult airway equipment immediately available.[2] Medications used for intubation combined with other traumatic injuries and positive pressure ventilation can produce hemodynamic instability and circulatory collapse. Nurses often assist in simultaneous resuscitation by administering fluids and blood products.[2,4]

During intubation, the nurse may be directed by the intubating provider to apply cricoid pressure, direct pressure on the anterior neck over the cricoid cartilage.[5] Cricoid pressure occludes the esophagus to decrease gastric distention during BVM and reduce aspiration risk but can also compromise the view of the larynx.[1,5] Once the endotracheal tube is placed, the nurse assists in confirming correct placement and securing the tube. Various methods can be used to secure the airway, such as tape, ties, straps, bite blocks, and specialty devices. While securement

---

Box 2
Nursing role in endotracheal intubation

Before Intubation
- Assist with patient position[1,5]
- Attach monitoring devices
  - EKG monitor
  - Pulse oximeter
  - Automatic blood pressure monitor
- Ensure preoxygenation
  - Administer high-flow oxygen
  - Assist with BVM if needed
- Gather and set up equipment[1]
  - Rigid suction device
  - BVM
  - Oropharyngeal and nasopharyngeal airways
  - Laryngoscope with various blades
  - Endotracheal tubes in various sizes
  - Lubricant o end-tidal CO2 detector
  - Securement device o gum-elastic bougie
  - Cricothyroidotomy kit (needle or surgical)
  - Video laryngoscope
- Check equipment function

During Intubation
- Administer intubation drugs as ordered
  - Rapid-acting and short-duration drugs preferred[5]
  - May include induction drugs, sedatives/hypnotics, opioids, paralytics[1]
- Apply cricoid pressure as directed[1]
- Monitoring with simultaneous resuscitation[1]
  After Intubation
- Assist with confirming tube placement[5]
  - Auscultation of bilateral lung fields and epigastrum
  - Observe condensation in tube
  - Ensure chest radiograph is ordered
- Assist with securing the tube[5]
- Continue monitoring vitals[1]
- Adjunct interventions[4]
  - Place orogastric tube as ordered
  - Restraints as needed
  - Analgesic and sedative administration

Abbreviation: EKG, electrocardiogram.

---

certain methods are preferred by institutions; none of the methods have proved to be superior to the others.[2]

Bedside nurses work closely with respiratory therapists to maintain a patent airway, prevent airway loss, clear secretions, avoid obstruction, and prevent infection.[2,10] Endotracheal tubes and tracheostomies should be kept secure to prevent unplanned removal or tube migration, microaspiration, and airway injury. Airway maintenance includes oral care, endotracheal tube and tracheostomy suctioning, subglottic suctioning, and cuff pressure management.[2,10]

TRAUMATIC AIRWAY INJURIES

Traumatic airway injury (TAI) involves lacerations, hematoma, fractures, or tears within the upper or lower airways. TAIs are relatively uncommon, occurring in 0.5% to 2% of blunt traumas and 1% to 6% of traumas with penetrating mechanism.[11] Injuries to the upper airway (above the cervical trachea) can occur from hyperextension of the neck, strangulation, and direct blows or penetration of the face or neck. Lower airway injuries below the cervical trachea can be caused by sudden deceleration or anterolateral chest compression. Increased intrathecal pressure against a closed glottis from blunt trauma to the neck, thorax, or abdomen can cause injury to both upper and lower airways.[11]

Up to 80% of patients with airway trauma die at the scene.[11,12] Prognosis of injury within the hospital setting depends on concomitant injuries, surgical requirements, and the amount of time to diagnosis and treatment. Lower airway injuries are usually occult in nature, leading to delayed recognition. Concomitant injuries can also cause delay in diagnosis of TAI, leading to increased mortality and complications such as hypoxia, airway stenosis, and recurrent pulmonary infections.[12] Oxygenation is more difficult when injuries are distal to the tip of the endotracheal tube.[11] Complications occur in approximately 25% of patients with TAI, including prolonged stay in the intensive care unit, surgical complications, airway stenosis, and problems with phonation.[12]

Diagnosis

Patients with TAI may present with dysphonia (hoarse voice), hemoptysis, subcutaneous emphysema, palpable laryngeal fracture, and respiratory distress.[11,12] Patients with lower airway injuries may have persistent hypoxemia after endotracheal intubation, persistent pneumothorax or air leak after chest tube placement, and significant pneumomediastinum.[11,12]

During the primary survey, chest radiograph may show signs of potential TAI. Subcutaneous emphysema can be seen in 87% of lower airway injuries.[11] Chest radiograph may also show pneumothorax, pneumomediastinum, or tracheal deformity.[11,12] With tracheal injury, the endotracheal tube may seem to protrude beyond the outline of the trachea.[11] However, 10% to 20% of patients with tracheobronchial injuries show no signs on radiograph.[12] Ultrasound performed in the trauma bay can help detect pneumothorax or subcutaneous emphysema.[11]

Computed tomography (CT) is commonly used for trauma workup and should be done on all patients with suspicion of TAI.[11] If cartilage fractures are suspected but not seen on CT scan, an MRI may be performed.[11] Patients with suspected or confirmed TAI should undergo bronchoscopy to locate the site of injury, verify the extent or depth, and ensure the cuff of the endotracheal tube is inflated beyond the site of injury.[12] Bronchoscopy may reveal tearing or lacerations, blood in the airway, or airway collapse.[11]

Treatment

In emergency situations, patients with an unstable airway or with obvious signs of airway injury should be intubated or have emergent operative intervention before imaging.[11] The endotracheal tube cuff should be inflated distal to the injury to avoid worsening the injury, pneumothorax, and subcutaneous emphysema.[12] Injuries of the upper airway are often addressed during airway triage, with definitive airway placement.[11] Minor injuries, such as mucosal flaps, nondisplaced laryngeal fractures, and small hematomas can be managed nonoperatively, whereas more serious injuries require surgical fixation. Treatment of upper airway injury focuses on restoring normal voice and swallowing.[11] Lower airway injuries often require surgery to close the defect, improve ventilation, and prevent spillage into the mediastinum.[11,12] Surgical methods may include direct repair with sutures, resection of the injured area, or partial pneumonectomy. Early surgical intervention generally leads to improved long-term outcomes.[12] Patients with TAI who are high risk for surgery due to comorbidities may undergo silicone or metallic stenting, which stay in place for 4 to 6 weeks.[11]

CASE STUDY

A 12-year-old boy with no significant past medical history was the front seat passenger involved in motor vehicle collision with airbag deployment against the neck and chest. He was brought to the emergency department by prehospital personnel in a cervical collar. Initial primary assessment showed increased work of breathing and inspiratory stridor. He was alert but unable to state his name on questioning. Subcutaneous emphysema was present in the anterior neck with small laceration not actively bleeding. Contusion was noted in the upper chest. Respiratory rate was 30 bpm with marked sternal recession, heart rate was 125 bpm (sinus tachycardia on the monitor), and blood pressure was 100/52 mmHg. Oxygen saturation was 90% on nonrebreather mask. Extremities were cool.

Acute laryngeal trauma was suspected. Airway triage was performed by senior emergency attending physician while awaiting arrival of the trauma team. Initially, jaw thrust maneuver was performed to open the airway and BVM was performed to support respirations. Respiratory status did not improve, and level of consciousness declined. RSI (orotracheal) was attempted under direct laryngoscopy but was unsuccessful. Jaw thrust maneuver again was performed and oropharyngeal airway was inserted. BVM ventilation was performed for approximately 3 minutes until oxygenation saturation increased to 100%. A second pass at orotracheal intubation was attempted, but oxygen saturations decreased rapidly to 70. The decision was made to perform a surgical cricothyroidotomy. After the endotracheal tube was inserted into the neck, bilateral breath sounds were auscultated, condensation was noted in the tube, and color change was noted on the carbon dioxide detector. Oxygen saturations improved to 96% on the mechanical ventilator. The tube was secured, and chest radiograph was done to confirm tube depth.

The child was retrieved by advanced care medical team within the hour and transported to tertiary children's hospital intensive care unit (ICU). A tracheostomy was performed in the Pediatric ICU, and his esophagus underwent surgical repair. The ventilator was weaned to a T-piece on day 5 and off oxygen on day 6. The patient remained hemodynamically stable. Intermittent cuff deflation was attempted on day 10. On day 16, the patient tolerated oral feeding and cuff deflation with good cough reflex. He was discharged from the ICU on day 20.

CLINICS CARE POINTS

- Airway is the first priority in trauma care.
- Airway assessment should be repeated frequently on trauma patients with risk of airway compromise.
- Cervical spine immobility is a major contributor to airway difficulty.
- The trauma team should always be prepared for a difficult airway, and adjunct equipment and staff should be readily available.
- Simultaneous resuscitation is often required due to hemodynamic instability.

DISCLOSURE STATEMENT

There are no commercial or financial conflicts of interests to disclose.

REFERENCES

1. American College of Surgeons Committee on Trauma. Advanced trauma Life support student course manual. 10th ed. American College of Surgeons; 2018.

2. Brown CVR, Inaba K, Shatz DV, et al. Western Trauma Association critical decisions in trauma: airway management in the adult trauma patients. J Trauma Acute Care Surg 2020;5:e000539. https://doi.org/10.1136/tsaco-2020-000539.
3. NurseEdu.com. Anatomy and physiology made easy. NEDU Publishing; 2021.
4. Kovacs G, Sowers N. Airway management in trauma. Emerg Med Clin North Am 2018;36:61–84. https://doi.org/10.1016/j.emc.2017.08.006.
5. Society of Critical Care Medicine. Fundamental critical care support. 7th edition. Society of Critical Care Medicine; 2021.
6. Merchant RM, Topjian AA, Panchal AR, et al. Part 1: Executive summary: 2020 American heart association guidelines for cardiopulmonary resuscitation and emergency cardiovascular care. Circulation (New York, N.Y.). 2020;142:S337–57.
7. Sheppard J, Coughenour JP, Barnes SL. Chapter 7: airway and perioperative management. In: Moore FD, Rhee PM, Rodriguez CJ, editors. Surgical and critical care and emergency surgery: Clinical questions and answers. 3rd edition. Wiley Blackwell; 2022. p. 67–76.
8. Sheikh F, Fox AD. Chapter 26: common procedures in the ICU. In: Moore FD, Rhee PM, Rodriguez CJ, editors. Surgical and critical care and emergency surgery: Clinical questions and answers. 3rd edition. Wiley Blackwell; 2022. p. 273–9.
9. Raschke E, Kobayashi L. Chapter 29: blunt and penetrating neck trauma. In: Moore FD, Rhee PM, Rodriguez CJ, editors. Surgical and critical care and emergency surgery: Clinical questions and answers. 3rd edition. Wiley Blackwell; 2022. p. 307–17.
10. Dexter AM, Scott JB. Airway management and ventilator-associated events. Respir Care 2019;64(8):986–93. https://doi.org/10.4187/respcare.07107.
11. Bagga B, Kumar A, Chahal A, et al. Traumatic airway injuries: role of imaging. Curr Probl Diagn Radiol 2020;49:48–53. https://doi.org/10.1067/j.cpradiol.2018.10.005.
12. Prokakis C, Koletsis EN, Dedeilias P, et al. Airway trauma: a review on epidemiology, mechanisms of injury, diagnosis, and treatment. J Card Surg 2014;9:117. https://doi.org/10.1186/1749-8090-9-117.

Acute Management of Cervical Spinal Cord Injuries

Alexandra Hunt, MSN, CRNP, AGACNP-BC*,
Karen A. McQuillan, MS, RN, CNS-BC, CCRN, CNRN, TCRN, FAAN

KEYWORDS

- Cervical spinal cord injury • American Spinal Injury Association • Neurogenic shock
- Spinal shock

KEY POINTS

- The goal of acute management is to prevent secondary injury to the cervical spinal cord.
- Cervical spinal cord injury impacts several organ systems of the body. It is important to have a regimented and systematic approach to care.
- Sufficient perfusion and oxygenation is essential to preventing secondary spinal cord injury.

INTRODUCTION

Cervical spinal cord injuries occur as a result of trauma that compresses, penetrates, impedes blood flow or causes shearing of the spinal cord below the brainstem to the cervical level 8 spinal nerve or from C1 to C7 vertebrae. The common causes of cervical spinal cord injury include car/motorcycle crashes, falls, violent acts (eg, stab wounds), and recreational injuries (eg, diving). Patients who sustain trauma to the cervical spine are most likely to suffer fracture/injury at C5–C7.[1] Hyperextension, hyperflexion, rotation, axial loading, distraction, and penetrating injuries are the common mechanisms responsible for the different fracture patterns of the cervical spine.[2]

According to the National Spinal Cord Injury Statistical Center, there are about 17,000 new spinal cord injuries each year in the United States.[3] Currently, in the United States, it is estimated that nearly 300,000 Americans have a spinal cord injury.[3] Men are more likely to be affected by spinal cord injury than women.[3] Historically, patients were younger; however, there has been an increase in average age of Americans with spinal cord injury. Men and women with spinal cord injury are more likely to be hospitalized in their lifetime and a have a higher mortality rate compared with patients with other injuries.[3] The most common causes of mortality in the spinal cord population include sepsis and pneumonia.[3]

R Adams Cowley Shock Trauma Center, University of Maryland Medical Center, 22 South Greene Street, Baltimore, MD 21201, USA
* Corresponding author.
E-mail address: alexandra.hunt@umm.edu

Crit Care Nurs Clin N Am 35 (2023) 119–128
https://doi.org/10.1016/j.cnc.2023.02.004
0899-5885/23/© 2023 Elsevier Inc. All rights reserved.

PATHOPHYSIOLOGY

Spinal cord injury can be divided into two phases: primary injury and secondary injury. Primary injury occurs at the moment that the initial injury to the spinal cord is sustained. This sets off a cascade of events at the cellular level which leads to cell death and scar formation on the spinal cord.[4] Prolonged cord compression leading to decreased blood flow and hypoxia of the injured spine can increase secondary spinal cord injury, thereby worsening neurologic outcome of the patient. The main goal of management for patients suffering from an acute spinal cord injury is to prevent secondary injury.

SPINAL AND NEUROGENIC SHOCK

Spinal shock, the acute loss of spinal function below the level of injury, begins at or near the moment of injury to the cervical spine. Ditunno and colleagues described a four-phase model of spinal shock which focuses on the impact of the injury on ones' reflexes.[5] See **Table 1** for further description of the phases.

In patients with spinal cord injury at or above the T6 level, the sympathetic nervous system can be cut off from the higher control centers in the brain, whereas the parasympathetic vagal nerve remains intact. This is results in a slowed heart rate and vasodilation, causing inadequate tissue perfusion, known as neurogenic shock. Neurogenic shock can be confounded by hemorrhagic shock on the initial presentation.

DIAGNOSIS

On arrival to a trauma center or emergency room, a patient suspected to have a spinal cord injury undergoes a trauma assessment according to the Advanced Trauma Life Support Guidelines.[6] The initial assessment focuses on the airway, breathing, and circulation while maintaining spinal precautions. These precautions include the placement of a cervical collar, maintenance of the head of bed flat, and the use of log roll with turns. Once the patient is stabilized, which may include stopping hemorrhage, intubation for airway protection and administration of fluids, vasopressors, or blood to achieve hemodynamic stability, the secondary assessment begins. The secondary assessment focuses on evaluation of any obvious deformity to the extremities, palpation of the entire spine, and an assessment of rectal tone. Ultrasound imaging for a Focused Assessment with Sonography in Trauma and initial x-rays occur as well. Computerized tomography (CT) scans are conducted to assess for any fractures or dislocations of the vertebrae. MRI is the preferred choice of imaging to assess for ligamentous injury, spinal cord edema, or cord compression.[2,7]

Table 1 Four phase model of spinal shock		
Phase	**Time Course Post-Injury**	**Description**
Phase 1	0–24 h	Loss of reflexes
Phase 2	1–3 d	Reflexes begin to return
Phase 3	4 d to 1 mo	Beginning of hyperreflexia
Phase 4	1–12 mo post-injury	Hyperreflexia and spasticity

From Ditunno, JF, Little, JW, Tessler, A et al. Spinal shock revisited: A four-phase model. *Spinal Cord*, 2004: 42(7), 383 to 395. https://doi.org/10.1038/sj.sc.3101603

A focused neurologic assessment is performed to determine sensory and motor function of the patient. The three nerve tracts typically assessed to determine spinal cord function are described in **Table 2**.

CASE PRESENTATION PART 1

AW was a 20-year-old woman who presented after diving into a shallow pool. She was unable to move her extremities and had decreased sensation below her nipple line. She had difficulty breathing with paradoxic abdominal movements. Her initial oxygen saturation was low at 90%. AW was intubated for airway protection. The initial heart rate was in the 50s, and blood pressure was 80s/60s. A liter of plasma-lyte was administered, and norepinephrine was started with noted improvement in her blood pressure. After undergoing CT imaging, AW was found to have a burst fracture at C5 with cord compression. She was taken to the operating room for decompression of her cervical spine and then admitted to the intensive care unit (ICU) for further management.

AMERICAN SPINAL INJURY ASSOCIATION SCALE

The American Spinal Injury Association (ASIA) created the International Standards for Neurologic Classification of Spinal Cord Injury assessment tool which assigns a numeric score for motor and sensory function and an alphabetical grade (A–E) to describe the extent of impairment below the level of injury.[8] The specific grade may help with the prognostication of the patient's likelihood for regaining function. The grades of ASIA Impairment Scale (AIS) are briefly reviewed below in **Table 3**. For a more detailed description of the tool, it can be accessed on the ASIA Web site (https://asia-spinalinjury.org).

CASE PRESENTATION PART 2

Once the patient, AW, was admitted to the ICU, an initial neurologic assessment was completed. For her motor score, she was able to shrug her shoulders and could contract her biceps on both upper extremities. Sensation was still noted to be above the nipple line. AW continued to participate in daily AIS examinations to determine her function postoperatively.

CLASSIFICATION OF INJURY

Spinal cord injuries are divided into two categories: complete and incomplete. Complete injury refers to the patient having no sensory or motor function below the level of

Table 2		
Nerve tracts typically assessed to determine spinal cord function		
Nerve Tracts Assessed	**Function of the Nerve Tracts**	**Technique Used for Assessment**
Lateral spinothalamic	Pain and temperature from the opposite side of the body	Assess ability to distinguish sharp vs dull sensory stimulation in each dermatome of the body on the right and left side
Posterior column	Proprioception, vibration, touch	Determine if the patient can sense the position of their digit moved up or down in each of the four extremities
Lateral corticospinal	Voluntary motor function	Assess strength of motor function in key muscles on the right and left side of the body

Table 3	
American Spinal Injury Association impairment scale	
Grade	**Description**
A	This is considered a complete injury. Motor or sensory function is not preserved below the level of injury
B	Motor function is not preserved below the level of injury; however, sensory function can be
C	Motor function is incomplete and less than half of the muscle groups have strength greater than or equal to three
D	Motor function is incomplete and at least half of the muscle groups have a strength greater than or equal to three
E	No sensory or motor deficits

Adapted from American Spinal Injury Association. International Standards for Neurological Classification of Spinal Cord Injury. https://asia-spinalinjury.org/wp-content/uploads/2019/10/ASIA-ISCOS-Worksheet_10.2019_PRINT-Page-1-2.pdf Accessed June 18, 2022.

injury. This correlates with an AIS grade A. Incomplete injury (AIS grade B–D) varies in regard to the amount of sensory or motor function the patient has below the level of injury. **Table 4** describes the common incomplete injury patterns or syndromes.

ACUTE MANAGEMENT

Timing of Decompression: The fracture pattern and whether there is spinal cord involvement dictate the type of surgical plan required for the patient. Surgical decompression has become a part of the treatment algorithm for acute spinal cord injury to prevent secondary injury as long as the patient is medically stable. The exact timing of surgery is important in regard to the impact it will have on the patient's neurologic outcome. The largest study looking at this timeline was the Surgical Timing in Acute Spinal Cord Injury Study. This multicenter study compared outcomes in patients who had surgical decompression performed in less than 24 hours to those decompressed greater than 24 hours after injury. The outcomes showed that there was a benefit in neurologic outcomes in the early surgical decompression group.[9] There

Table 4	
Incomplete spinal cord injuries	
Type of Injury	**Description**
Central cord	Greater motor function loss in the upper extremities than in the lower extremities; Sensory loss is variable.
Brown-Sequard syndrome	Loss of motor function and proprioception on the injured side at and below the level of spinal cord injury; Loss of pain and temperature sensation on the opposite side of the body at and below the level of injury.
Anterior cord syndrome	Loss of motor function, pain and touch at and below the level of injury. Proprioception and vibration sensation remain intact.
Posterior cord syndrome	No decline in motor function or pain and temperature sensation; Only loss of proprioception and vibration sensation.

Data from Refs[7,10,21]

continues to be more trials that further investigate the most appropriate timing for surgical fixation and the impact it has on the neurologic outcome after spinal cord injury.

Pain: After injury to the cervical spine, patients may have intense pain especially in the neck and shoulders. A multimodal approach should be used to relieve that pain. Medications that may be used include opioids, non-opiate analgesics, nonsteroidal anti-inflammatory, anti-spasmodic agents, and drugs to treat neuropathic pain.[10] Spasticity is a complication which may continue well after the acute period and is also treated with range of motion, muscle stretching, proper positioning, and splinting.[11]

Respiratory

Individuals who have sustained a cervical spinal cord injury are at high risk for respiratory failure. Depending on the level of injury, the patient's muscles used for respiration and secretion clearance can be paralyzed. The diaphragm is innervated by the phrenic nerve at the C3–C5 level. [12,13] Patients with cervical spinal cord injury will primarily use their diaphragm to breath and will appear to have a paradoxic breathing pattern, where the abdomen is moving in the opposite direction of the chest wall. This is known as quad breathing.[2] Impaired respiratory mechanics put the patient at high risk for atelectasis and hypercapnia. Due to the paralysis of muscles used to cough, secretion clearance will be poor therefore increasing the risk of pneumonia. In the ICU, it is important that patients with cervical spinal injury be placed on a regimented secretion clearance pathway using mucolytics, chest physiotherapy, cough assist, and intrapulmonary percussive ventilation. Nursing staff may assist a patient with coughing by placing a folded towel or blanket on the upper abdomen and using his or her hand on the towel or blanket to push upwards toward the chest during the patient's exhalation.[12]

If the patient has a high cervical spine lesion, there is a high likelihood that a tracheostomy will be needed to possibly liberate from the mechanical ventilator. Research has been conducted on the appropriate timing of tracheostomy for patients with cervical spinal cord injury. Early tracheostomy may decrease the length of time that the patient is in the ICU and time on the ventilator.[12–14]

When patients can start weaning from the ventilator, it is important to monitor for signs of tachypnea and the use of accessory muscles. They may easily tire from the respiratory exercises, leading to the development of atelectasis and hypercapnia. End-tidal carbon dioxide monitoring or the collection of arterial blood gas should be considered to monitor the level of carbon dioxide in the blood.[15] Some patients with high cervical spine fractures may not be able to wean from the ventilator. A rigorous respiratory regimen should be continued to help with secretion clearance and the prevention of pneumonia. If the patient's phrenic nerve is intact, one may be a candidate to have a diaphragmatic pacer placed. Diaphragmatic pacing has been found to help patients wean off the ventilator.[16]

Respiratory failure is one of the main causes of cardiopulmonary arrest among patients with spinal cord injury. It can be precipitated by a drop in oxygen level, followed by bradycardia. It is important to administer an agent to elevate heart rate and to assist the patient with ventilation with administration of supplemental oxygen to quickly improve oxygenation. The patient may require a therapeutic bronchoscopy to support secretion clearance.[15] If an incidence like this occurs, it is important to readjust the patient's mucolytics and to investigate other medical sources for this event.

Cardiovascular

Mean Arterial Pressure Push: Sufficient blood pressure must be maintained to prevent secondary injury by promoting ample blood flow to the injured spinal cord. In order to do this, the patients mean arterial pressure (MAP) is elevated as able depending on the patients' baseline cardiac function. The American Association of Neurologic Surgeons/Congress of Neurologic Surgeons suggests that the MAP should be augmented to 85 to 90 mm Hg for the first 7 days after a spinal cord injury.[17] It is important to ensure that adequate intravascular volume is established. Medications which may be used to augment the blood pressure include norepinephrine, epinephrine, dopamine, and midodrine.[18]

Bradycardia: After spinal cord injury at and above T6, bradycardia can occur contributing to neurogenic shock. This necessitates continuous monitoring of the patient's heart rate and rhythm. Different treatment modalities have been studied to determine safe and effective options for treating bradycardia. Enteric albuterol has been found to safely treat bradycardia associated with spinal cord injury.[19] Another enteric medication is theophylline.[20] Intravenous medications such as epinephrine, atropine, or dobutamine may be used as well to treat symptomatic bradycardia. [20]

Orthostatic Hypotension: After cervical spinal cord injury, the loss of sympathetic control often causes orthostatic hypotension when the patient is placed in a head-up or seated position. It is recommended to wrap patients' legs in compression stockings and ace bandages before getting out of bed and to gradually raise the head in order to maintain a normal blood pressure.[21,22] Midodrine, an alpha-adrenergic agonist that increases vascular tone and blood pressure, can also be administered to help prevent or treat orthostatic hypotension.[23]

CASE PRESENTATION PART 3

AW underwent the recommended MAP push. She was started on around-the-clock midodrine to decrease the amount of norepinephrine needed to maintain her blood pressure. Also, she was started on around-the-clock albuterol to avoid bradycardia. After 7 days, her MAP goal was liberalized to 65 mm Hg or greater. She remained on midodrine; however, it was weaned as able to support her blood pressure at the new liberalized MAP goal.

During the first week of her stay in the ICU, she was weaned to pressure support ventilation from a rate on the ventilator. She was noted to have a weak cough and had a moderate amount of slightly thick secretions. She was placed on short spontaneous breathing trials with decreased ventilator settings to assess the possibility of extubation. Ascending edema was noted on her postoperative MRI, so the decision was made to proceed with performing a tracheostomy. The tracheostomy procedure was uncomplicated. She began an organized trach collar trial regimen to wean from the ventilator. Her young age and active life style before her injury assisted her progress with ventilator weaning.

Temperature Management

Due to disruption of the sympathetic nervous system from its higher control centers patients with cervical spinal cord injury lose the ability to control their body temperature. Body temperature can vary depending on the environment; known as poikilothermia.[15] This phenomenon necessitates that the patient's body temperature be monitored continuously or frequently and interventions are used to warm or cool the patient to maintain normothermia. One simple thing a nurse can do is to monitor the temperature in the patient's room and adjust it accordingly to maintain the patient's desired body temperature. It is not uncommon for a patient with spinal cord injury to be febrile after injury. It is important to consider infectious sources (eg, pneumonia and urinary tract infections), drug fever, and atelectasis as other possible sources which may cause the patient's fever.

Nutrition

After acute spinal cord injury, patients are typically in a high catabolic state, necessitating attention to ensure adequate nutrition is provided. As the patient progresses, a swallow evaluation may be performed due to high risk of dysphagia with this patient population. Risk factors for dysphagia include high cervical spinal cord injury, anterior cervical surgeries, and the presence of a tracheostomy.[24] It is important to have a speech pathologist assess patients on their ability to swallow post-injury before advancing the diet. A surgical feeding tube should be considered in patients who fail the swallow study or when there is concern for insufficient oral intake to meet adequate nutrition needs.

CASE PRESENTATION PART 4

When liberalized from the ventilator, a speech pathologist was consulted to assist with a speaking valve. AW was very excited to hear her voice while using the speaking valve. A swallow evaluation was conducted which she failed initially. On her second evaluation, she passed for a modified diet and eventually was able to progress to a regular diet with thin liquids.

Bowel and Bladder Function

Patients with spinal cord injury suffer from bladder and bowel dysfunction. Those with cervical spinal cord injury typically have stool retention during spinal shock and then hyper-reflexive bowel once spinal shock resolves. With a hyper-reflexive bowel, there is no sensation or control of defecation due to a spastic external sphincter and reflexive stool propulsion.[25] It is important to promote a stringent bowel regimen that promotes soft-formed stool that can be evacuated at regular intervals. Common medications used are stool softeners, laxatives, and suppositories.[7,25] Patients with spinal cord injury are at risk for ileus which should be readily recognized to avoid abdominal distension and possible aspiration of enteric feedings.[7]

High cervical spinal cord injury patients who are in spinal shock will have urinary retention. After spinal shock resolves, the patient will have a reflexive bladder with spontaneous voiding at low volumes. A bladder training regimen helps with prevention of bladder distension and overflow. After bladder catheter removal, frequent intermittent catheterization can be initiated to empty the bladder.[7,25] Nurses can help patients with timing oral fluid intake around straight catheterizations to prevent bladder distension. If a patient starts to void, post-void residuals should be checked to determine whether the patient is experiencing overflow.

Immobility

Deep Vein Thrombosis: Immobility associated with cervical spinal cord injury puts patients at high risk for developing deep vein thromboses (DVTs). To prevent the formation of DVT, subcutaneous heparin or enoxaparin and pneumatic compression devices are used during the acute management period. Ideally, DVT prophylaxis will be initiated within 72 hours of injury.[21] Inferior Vena Cava filters have not shown benefit in the prevention of DVTs.[21]

Skin: Decreased sensation and immobility put individuals with spinal cord injury at risk for pressure injuries. Patients with high cervical spinal cord injury are three times more likely than those with lower spinal cord injury to develop a pressure ulcer and 14 times more likely to have a pressure ulcer compared with other patients who have sustained traumatic injuries.[26] Pressure injuries often occur in the sacral region, bony surfaces, and skin under cervical collars and endotracheal tube holders. Ways to prevent pressure injuries include frequent turning/repositioning, ensuring good stabilization device fit and using specialized pressure-relief mattresses and seat cushions. Nurses should perform thorough integument assessments and provide regular skin care including beneath cervical collars or other stabilization devices. If there is an area noted to be concern for skin breakdown, a wound specialist consult should be placed.[21]

Psychosocial Factors

Patients who sustain cervical spinal cord injuries often experience grief, depression, and frustration.[27] Their overall affect may become flat as they realize the implications of their injury on their future. Current research is targeted on determining different treatment methods to help with grief and depression after injury. One study suggests mindfulness activities may have beneficial outcomes.[28] It is recommended to have a strong family presence to support the patient. To help promote some control for the patient's situation, the nurse should include the patient in planning out the day (ie, the timing of getting out of bed, daily bath).[15] The lack of speech during intubation and mobility seem to be some of the most frustrating aspects of spinal cord injury. Physical and occupational therapy and speech pathologists should be consulted to help patients with these limitations.[21] Other resources which may be beneficial to both the patient and family include social work, chaplaincy, and support groups.[21]

CASE PRESENTATION PART 5

AW was discharged to an acute rehabilitation facility which specialized in neurologic injury. She completed her rehabilitation period and was able to return home with family.

CLINICAL PEARLS

- Ensure sufficient blood pressure and oxygenation to avoid secondary injury.
- Treat pain with at multimodal approach, which may include: non-pharmacologic interventions, opioids, non-opiate analgesics, nonsteroidal anti-inflammatories, antispasmodic agents, and drugs to treat neuropathic pain.
- Patients with spinal cord injury require a stringent respiratory protocol to promote secretion clearance.
- Prevent pressure ulcers by frequent repositioning of the patient.

DISCLOSURES

There are no commercial or financial disclosures for this article.

REFERENCES

1. Okereke I, Mmerem K, Balasubramanian D. The management of cervical spine injuries- A literature review. Orthop Res Rev 2021;13:151–61.
2. Rabinstein AA. Traumatic spinal cord injury. Continuum (Minneap Minn) 2018; 24(2):551–66. https://doi.org/10.1212/CON.0000000000000581. Spinal Cord Disorders).

3. National Spinal Cord Injury Statistical Center. Spinal Cord Injury and Figures at a Glance. University of Alabama at Birmingham: Birmingham, AL; 2020. Available at: http://www.nscisc.uab.edu/Public/Facts%20and%20Figures%202020.pdf. Accessed June 18, 2022.

4. Alizadeh A, Dyck SM, Karimi-Abdolrezaee S. Traumatic spinal cord injury: an overview of pathophysiology, models and acute injury mechanisms. Front Neurol 2019;10:282.

5. Ditunno JF, Little JW, Tessler A, et al. Spinal shock revisited: a four-phase model. Spinal Cord 2004;42(7):383–95.

6. American College of Surgeons Committee on Trauma. Advanced trauma life support student course manual. 10th ed. Chicago, IL: Author; 2018.

7. Wang TY, Park C, Zhang H, et al. Management of acute traumatic spinal cord injury: a review of the literature. Front Surg 2021;8:698736.

8. American Spinal Injury Association. International Standards for neurological classification of spinal cord injury. Available at: https://asia-spinalinjury.org/wp-content/uploads/2019/10/ASIA-ISCOS-Worksheet_10.2019_PRINT-Page-1-2.pdf. Accessed June 18, 2022.

9. Fehlings MG, Vaccaro A, Wilson JR, et al. Early versus delayed decompression for traumatic cervical spinal cord injury: results of the Surgical Timing in Acute Spinal Cord Injury Study (STASCIS). PLoS One 2012;7(2):e32037.

10. Hills TE. Caring for patients with a traumatic spinal cord injury. Nursing 2020; 50(12):30–40.

11. Nair KP, Marsden J. The management of spasticity in adults. BMJ 2014;349: g4737.

12. Schilero GJ, Bauman WA, Radulovic M. Traumatic spinal cord injury: pulmonary physiologic principles and management. Clin Chest Med 2018;39(2):411–25.

13. Mubashir T, Arif AA, Ernest P, et al. Early versus late tracheostomy in patients with acute traumatic spinal cord injury: a systematic review and meta-analysis. Anesth Analg 2021;132(2):384–94.

14. Khan M, Prabhakaran K, Jehan F, et al. Early tracheostomy in patients with cervical spine injury reduces morbidity and improves resource utilization. Am J Surg 2020;220(3):773–7.

15. Russo McCourt T. Spinal cord injuries. In: McQuillan KA, Flynn Makic MB, editors. Trauma nursing: from resuscitation through rehabilitation. 5th ed. St. Louis, MO: Elsevier; 2020. p. 454–502.

16. Posluszny JA Jr, Onders R, Kerwin AJ, et al. Multicenter review of diaphragm pacing in spinal cord injury: successful not only in weaning from ventilators but also in bridging to independent respiration. J Trauma Acute Care Surg 2014; 76(2):303–10.

17. Ryken TC, Hurlbert RJ, Hadley MN, et al. The acute cardiopulmonary management of patients with cervical spinal cord injuries. Neurosurgery 2013;72(Suppl 2):84–92.

18. Lee YS, Kim KT, Kwon BK. Hemodynamic management of acute spinal cord injury: a literature review. Neurospine 2021;18(1):7–14.

19. Lim-Hing K, Massetti J, Pajoumand M, et al. Impact of enteral albuterol on bradycardic events after acute cervical spinal cord injury. Neurocrit Care 2022;36(3): 840–5.

20. Perrine JA, Barber J, McKnight RL, et al. Theophylline for spinal cord injury associated bradycardia. J Pharm Pract 2022. https://doi.org/10.1177/0897190 0211064701. 8971900211064701.

21. American College of Surgeons. Best practices Guidelines spine injury. Chicago IL. 2021. Available at: https://www.facs.org/media/k45gikqv/spine_injury_guidelines.pdf. Accessed June 18 2022.

22. Hachem LD, Ahuja CS, Fehlings MG. Assessment and management of acute spinal cord injury: from point of injury to rehabilitation. J Spinal Cord Med 2017;40(6): 665–75.

23. Palma JA, Kaufmann H. Management of orthostatic hypotension. Continuum (Minneap Minn) 2020;26(1):154–77.

24. Hayashi T, Fujiwara Y, Ariji Y, et al. Mechanism of dysphagia after acute traumatic cervical spinal cord injury. J Neurotrauma 2020;37(21):2315–9.

25. Kuris EO, Alsoof D, Osorio C, et al. Bowel and bladder care in patients with spinal cord injury. J Am Acad Orthop Surg 2022;30(6):263–72.

26. Grigorian A, Sugimoto M, Joe V, et al. Pressure ulcer in trauma patients: a higher spinal cord injury level leads to higher risk. J Am Coll Clin Wound Spec 2018; 9(1–3):24–31.e1.

27. Klyce DW, Bombardier CH, Davis TJ, et al. Distinguishing grief from depression during acute recovery from spinal cord injury. Arch Phys Med Rehabil 2015;96(8): 1419–25.

28. Hearn JH, Cross A. Mindfulness for pain, depression, anxiety, and quality of life in people with spinal cord injury: a systematic review. BMC Neurol 2020;20(1):32.

Evidence-Based Pearls
Chest Trauma

Eleanor R. Fitzpatrick, DNP, RN, AGCNS-BC, ACNP-BC, CCRN, CCCTM

KEYWORDS

- Flail chest • Chest/thoracostomy tube • Emergency department thoracotomy (EDT)
- Damage control surgery and resuscitation • Thoracic endovascular aortic repair
- Pneumothorax • Hemothorax

KEY POINTS

- Thoracic trauma carries a high level of morbidity and mortality. It requires rapid, accurate assessments for abnormalities and pointed diagnostic testing to devise an effective management strategy.
- Surgeons may use damage control techniques to minimize the length of the initial surgical intervention to thwart the development of the deadly triad of hypothermia, acidosis, and coagulopathy.
- The elderly are at greater risk to sustain significant injury from varied mechanisms causing thoracic trauma. They are also more likely to develop trauma-related complications.

BACKGROUND AND INTRODUCTION

Historically, chest trauma had been an entity seen in wartime and now, in civilian life, young members of our society are most often affected. Traumatic injuries to the chest are one of the most common areas affected by both blunt and penetrating mechanisms. Blunt injury represents the most frequently seen type of chest trauma, associated with approximately 80% to 90% of injuries. Penetrating trauma is responsible for approximately 10% to 20% of thoracic injuries.[1–3]

Chest injuries are commonly seen in patients with polytrauma. Rapid identification and interventions are necessary to gain control of injuries to prevent the potentially life-threatening complications from worsening of the initial tissue damage.[3] This is especially true for the elderly population who are at risk for instability and complications due to reduced tolerance to injury at lower levels of force.[4] Older patients with systolic blood pressure less than 90 mm Hg after thoracic trauma have been found to be more vulnerable to complications and poor outcomes than their younger counterparts.[3,5]

Significant morbidity and mortality have accompanied thoracic trauma since its first description. In the United States, 25% to 35% of trauma-related deaths are due to

Surgical Intensive Care Unit, Thomas Jefferson University Hospital, Room 4465 Gibbon, 111 South 11th Street, Philadelphia, PA 19107, USA
E-mail address: Eleanor.fitzpatrick@jefferson.edu

Crit Care Nurs Clin N Am 35 (2023) 129–144
https://doi.org/10.1016/j.cnc.2023.02.005
0899-5885/23/© 2023 Elsevier Inc. All rights reserved.

thoracic trauma.[6] This level of morbidity and mortality is related to the disruption of respiration, circulation, or both. Respiratory decompensation develops from injury to the thoracic cage, lung parenchyma, or airways, which ultimately causes abnormalities in breathing. Altered pulmonary compliance leads to a ventilation-perfusion mismatch with hypoventilation and hypoxia. Deterioration in circulation is due to bleeding, impaired venous return, or injury to the heart. Regardless of the mechanism, bleeding within the thorax results in a hemothorax, which, if massive, will result in hypotension and hemorrhagic shock.[1,3,7] Operative intervention is required in approximately 10% patients with blunt injury to the thorax and 15% to 20% patients with penetrating chest injuries.[8]

Traumatic chest injuries can result from blunt or penetrating mechanisms to the thoracic cavity and/or chest wall. Blunt mechanisms include the following:

- Motor vehicle crashes (MVCs)
- Falls
- Pedestrians struck by vehicles
- Violent acts
- Blast injuries

Penetrating injuries to the chest are due to the use of guns and stabbing instruments. A rapid analysis of the extent of injury is critical to determine life-threatening injuries requiring immediate interventions.[1-3,6] **Table 1** delineates those injuries to the thorax, which are potentially lethal and those that are considered dangerous.

TYPES OF THORACIC INJURIES

The structures of the chest that can be injured in a traumatic event include the rib cage, chest wall, lung parenchyma, and visceral and parietal pleura. Mediastinal structures that can be disrupted by a traumatic mechanism include the heart, aorta, other major vessels, trachea, and esophagus. Many of these injuries occur in the setting of other equally severe injuries in polytrauma victims.[3]

Rib Fractures

The most commonly injured structure in the thoracic cavity is the ribs, which are most often fractured due to blunt trauma, especially in the elderly population.[4] Rib fractures are found in 85% of patients with chest trauma.[3] A significant amount of force is required to fracture ribs, particularly the 3 upper ribs. These ribs are protected by the musculature of the upper arms and when they are fractured, this is a marker for

Table 1 Lethal and Dangerous Thoracic Injuries	
Lethal and Dangerous Thoracic Injuries	
Lethal Scenarios	**Dangerous Scenarios**
Airway obstruction	Pulmonary contusion
Open pneumothorax	Myocardial contusion
Tension pneumothorax	Aortic disruption
Massive hemothorax	Diaphragmatic injury
Flail chest	Tracheobronchial tree disruption
Cardiac tamponade	Esophageal injury

Adapted from: Mert, Ü, Andruszkow, H & Hildebrand, F. Chest Trauma. In: Pape, H.C., editor. Textbook of Polytrauma Management, 3rd edition. Springer; 2022. p. 161 – 184.

severe concomitant injury. The energy required to cause rib fractures can be transmitted to underlying tissues resulting in damage such as pulmonary contusions and vascular disruption.[2,3] The lung parenchyma can be punctured by fractured ribs or by penetrating force, resulting in a pneumothorax (air escaping from the lung injury) or a hemothorax (blood escaping from injured blood vessels). The parenchyma of the lung can also be contused or lacerated from a traumatic mechanism.

The number of ribs fractured has a strong connection to the severity of injury and associated mortality. The mortality rate for patients admitted with rib fractures is approximately 10% but increases with each additional rib fracture and can be as high as 40% if more than 6 ribs are fractured. Since the rib cage and chest wall are highly innervated by nerves, thoracic injuries are associated with a great deal of pain. When pain is not well controlled, complications can ensue due to splinting, difficulty ventilating, or eliminating secretions.[2]

Other complications associated with the pain of rib fractures include atelectasis, acute respiratory distress syndrome (ARDS), and pulmonary embolism. These complications increase the morbidity and mortality associated with rib fractures.

Flail Chest and Sternal Fracture

Flail chest occurs due to a specific rib fractures pattern defined as the fracture of 2 or more consecutive ribs in 2 or more places (**Fig. 1**).[3] This results in instability of the chest wall with a free-floating segment of chest wall with paradoxical chest wall movements. The chest wall pulls in with inspiration and out during expiration.[3]

Fractures to the sternum require a significant amount of energy, potentially causing concurrent pulmonary and myocardial injuries. Patients with chest wall injuries experience similar symptoms as patients with rib fractures and are at risk for the same pulmonary complications; therefore, the diagnostic testing, nursing and medical interventions are similar to those used with rib fractures.

The significance of flail chest and sternal fractures is not the fractures themselves but the injury to the underlying tissues, lungs, heart, vessels, or other structures.

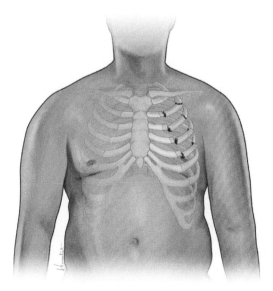

Fig. 1. Flail chest.

Most patients with flail chest or sternal fracture are managed with conservative, supportive therapy such as intensive pain management. In some cases, a sternal fracture may require passive reduction in the emergency department if the fracture is displaced.

Pneumothorax

A pneumothorax is the accumulation of air between the parietal and visceral pleura, which can result in a partial or total collapse of the lung. A simple pneumothorax neither expands during inspiration nor does it shift mediastinal structures as does a tension pneumothorax. Symptoms include shortness of breath, loss of breath sounds on one side, and subcutaneous tissue emphysema due to pleural lacerations from rib fractures or penetrating mechanism.[1,3,9]

When air in the lung cannot escape the cavity, a tension pneumothorax can develop due to the increasing positive pressure within the pleural space. This results in a collapse of the ipsilateral lung with compression and shift of mediastinal structures and the contralateral lung. The increased intrathoracic pressure results in dangerously reduced venous return to the heart with the potential for cardiovascular collapse. If a tension pneumothorax is suspected with signs of dyspnea, air hunger, distended jugular veins, unilateral breath sounds, and subcutaneous emphysema, the lung must be decompressed by needle thoracostomy. This is performed through the second intercostal space, midclavicular line anteriorly followed by the placement of a thoracostomy tube.[2,6,9] The Committee on Trauma of the American College of Surgeons has suggested that the fourth or fifth intercostal space between mid/anterior axillary line is the preferred area for decompression, although both approaches are included in the recommendation.[6,10] All trauma patients should be evaluated for a tension pneumothorax during the primary survey, and this should be considered should a patient begin to deteriorate unexpectedly.[2,6]

An open pneumothorax is a rare injury, also known as a "sucking" chest wound, which is a large opening in the chest wall due to a blast. When an affected patient inspires, air enters the lung through this opening rather than through the normal passage via the tracheobronchial tree.[1,6]

Hemothorax

A hemothorax develops when blood drains into the pleural cavity due to an injured vessel, such as an intercostal or internal mammary artery, or due to a direct injury to the heart. Patients may experience respiratory symptoms resulting from the size of the hemothorax and volume of lung space it occupies. Patients may also be hemodynamically unstable due to the blood loss and develop tachycardia and hypotension.[1] A massive hemothorax is considered the presence of 1500 mL of blood on placement of a thoracostomy tube or continued bleeding during the subsequent 2 to 4 hours.[1,11]

Pulmonary Contusion

Pulmonary contusion, injury to the lung parenchyma, is one of the most common injuries seen in patients with thoracic trauma. Pulmonary contusions can occur with direct impact to pulmonary structures, a deceleration episode, or with penetrating force and are found in 30% to 75% of patients sustaining thoracic trauma.[12] The contusion is caused by injured vasculature and tissues leaking blood and fluid into alveolar and interstitial spaces. These injuries are usually managed conservatively; patients are monitored closely for blossoming of the contusion and worsening pulmonary status with signs of complications, such as pneumonia and ARDS.[3] Patients who sustain a pulmonary laceration will always have a concomitant contusion. These patients are at even greater risk of developing ARDS due to the exaggerated inflammatory response from damage to the alveolar capillary membrane.[8,13]

Heart and Great Vessel Injuries

Cardiac injuries range in severity from simple contusion to laceration or rupture and are among the leading causes of death from trauma.[14] Severe penetrating wounds to the chest that damage the heart or the great vessels (aorta, superior vena cava, pulmonary veins) can also result in significant prehospital morbidity and mortality. Many patients succumb at the scene, although improved trauma transport systems have increased the number of patients successfully transported to hospitals.[9] Critical structures are within the "cardiac box," an area located between the nipples from sternal notch to xiphoid process (**Fig. 2**). Penetrating wounds to the mediastinum are markers for severe injury. Clinicians should have a high index of suspicion for cardiac injury in patients who sustain thoracic trauma, especially if it occurs within the cardiac box.[1,14]

Blunt injury to the heart and great vessels can occur from multiple causes. During MVCs, blunt cardiac injury can result from abrupt deceleration on impact with the steering wheel or dashboard. This type of blunt force can cause disruption of the heart or the descending thoracic aorta at its attachment to the ligamentum arteriosum with resultant bleeding.[1,2,15] Myocardial contusions are the most common injuries to the heart following blunt trauma, most commonly occurring from MVC, falls, assaults, and sports injuries where the heart strikes the sternum and anterior chest wall.[2] The spectrum of injury severity of myocardial contusions ranges from subepicardial/subendocardial bruising to full thickness necrosis with impaired cardiac function and cardiogenic shock. Myocardial rupture, valve rupture, and coronary artery dissection can also occur.[2] The highest incidence of myocardial contusion is due to MVC, falls, assaults, and sporting injuries whereby the heart strikes the sternum and anterior chest wall.[2]

The most common characteristic of myocardial contusions are arrhythmias, including tachycardias, atrial arrhythmias, and conduction abnormalities. The need for hospitalization and close monitoring is based on the presence of arrhythmias and hemodynamic stability. Unexplained shock or hypotension in a patient who experiences significant high-energy impact or deceleration should result in further

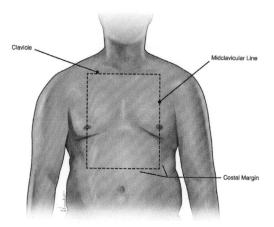

Clavicle

Midclavicular Line

Costal Margin

Fig. 2. The "Cardiac Box".

diagnostic testing to exclude blunt cardiac injury.[16] Other clinical indicators of potential blunt cardiac injury include Beck's triad of hypotension, distended jugular venous distension, and muffled heart sounds or evidence of a hemothorax and refractory hypotension. A missed injury due to this mechanism can result in significant morbidity and mortality.[15,17,18]

Cardiac tamponade occurs most frequently with stab wounds and gunshot wounds (GSW) to the chest. Injured vessels bleed into an intact pericardial sac, and this compresses the atria, impairing venous return and cardiac filling. Patients may present in extremis or they may be alert but hypotensive and exhibit extreme anxiety. Beck's triad may also occur but is a rare finding. The diagnosis of this injury must be made quickly because deterioration and cardiovascular collapse are imminent.[1–3] Traumatic cardiac rupture most commonly affects the right ventricle due to its anterior location in the chest. The thin wall of the right ventricle also contributes to the potential for rupture.

Most thoracic great vessel injuries (vena cava, aorta, pulmonary veins) are caused by penetrating external mechanisms such as GSW. Blunt causes for major vessel disruption include high-speed head-on or side-impact collision. The most commonly injured vessels are the descending thoracic aorta, innominate artery, pulmonary veins, and vena cava.[15,19] Traumatic aortic injuries are seen in a small percentage of those with chest trauma but are life-threatening. The most common cause of traumatic aortic injuries is blunt force. In approximately 90% of cases, those with complete aortic rupture succumb at the scene of the traumatic incident, commonly a high-speed MVC.[19] Patients only survive due to the development of an adherent clot or other condition, which contains active bleeding.[3,15]

Other Mediastinal Injuries

Esophageal injuries are rare and occur mostly from penetrating trauma.[3] Patients that present after penetrating trauma with a hemothorax or pneumothorax without rib fracture or those that sustain a severe blow to the chest should be closely examined for signs of esophageal injury. Failure to diagnose this injury can be lethal, resulting in spillage of esophageal contents and mediastinitis. Pleural effusion is commonly associated with esophageal disruption and particulate matter may be present in chest tube drainage.[9] Patients may present with pain or shock out of proportion to clinical findings. Once identified, surgery is necessary to repair the esophagus and antibiotics should be given to prevent mediastinitis.[3,9,20] Other complications after esophageal injury include stenosis, fistula, wound infection, and pneumonia.[20]

Tracheobronchial injuries occur rarely, primarily due penetrating trauma or to crushing/compressive force to the thorax, which tears or lacerates the trachea or bronchi. These injuries are often associated with esophageal, pulmonary, or vascular injury.[3,9] Patients present with a range of symptoms from severe respiratory distress secondary to airway compromise, hemoptysis, or airway obstruction. An early sign of an injury to the trachea or mainstem bronchi is a pneumothorax, initially managed with thoracostomy tube insertion but with rapidly developing bronchopleural air leaks requiring additional tubes. Identifying these injuries and stabilizing the airway and hemodynamic status are keys to improved outcomes.[3]

DIAGNOSTIC TESTING

Injuries to the chest wall may be identified with physical examination and chest radiograph. An initial chest radiograph is recommended after blunt thoracic trauma unless minor and the patient has no signs of potential injury.[1,3,7] In patients with significant thoracic trauma experiencing shortness of breath or unilateral decreased or absent breath sounds, a pneumothorax or hemothorax should be presumed and no diagnostic studies are indicated. A thoracostomy tube should be inserted. In patients who are hemodynamically stable computed tomography (CT) with contrast will identify injuries.[9] Small pneumothoraces may go undiagnosed and additional diagnostic testing may be required once the patient has been stabilized.

Stable patients may be candidates for a computed tomography angiogram (CTA) to identify missile trajectory and reveal injuries to underlying structures. A CTA is recommended for patients with polytrauma with suspected chest trauma and those with abnormal results of initial chest radiograph.[1,9] If identified, vascular injuries can be treated angiographically or surgically. Angiography may be used in cases in which CTA results are questionable or if images are unclear.[3,9]

Thoracic ultrasound or point of care ultrasound, a noninvasive diagnostic test that is efficient and generally available, provides information regarding the presence of trauma-related organ injury.

An Extended Focused Abdominal Sonography in Trauma (EFAST) examination may be performed to examine the chest wall and underlying organs. This test uses bedside ultrasound to identify pneumothorax, hemothorax, and other injuries.[1,21] These tests are used in conjunction with chest radiography because ultrasound is not sensitive or specific in the detection of bony injuries.[3,6] Additional injury-specific diagnostic tests are listed is in **Box 1**.

Scoring systems exist for determining the severity of thoracic trauma and for identifying appropriate diagnostic management strategies.[3,8] These scoring systems are based on altered physiologic parameters and include the Abbreviated Injury Scale, Thoracic Abbreviated Injury Score, Pulmonary Contusion Scale, CT-Dependent Wagner Score, and Thoracic Trauma Severity Score.[1] Assessing the severity of traumatic thoracic injuries can provide a great deal of information early in the course of the post-injury period. They can provide clinicians an accurate index of suspicion for the development of complications or mortality in these patients. Accurately identifying the severity of injury can aid physicians and nurses in insuring that patients in need are appropriately admitted to critical care units if indicated and receive evidence-based

---

Box 1
Injury-Specific Diagnostic Tests

Injury-Specific Diagnostic Tests

Esophageal trauma
- Radiograph reveals mediastinal air, pleural effusion
- CT esophagography or CT
- Esophagoscopy
    Tracheobronchial injuries
    - Radiograph reveals mediastinal air
    - Bronchoscopy-gold standard for diagnosis
    Myocardial contusions and other cardiac injuries
    - Electrocardiogram—if normal, blunt injury still possible
    - Chest radiograph
    - Cardiac troponin-reliable for myocardial cell damage
    - Transthoracic echocardiogram identifies abnormal contractility
    - Transesophageal echo
    - CT
    - EFAST
    - MRI—limited role due to availability and timeliness[17,22]

interventions. More exploration is needed with these scoring systems to enhance their accuracy, speed, and ease of use and to increase their universal applicability.[3,8]

MANAGEMENT OF THORACIC INJURIES

Patients experiencing thoracic trauma should be managed in accordance with the ABCDE algorithm of the Advanced Trauma Life Support guidelines that address airway control (A), breathing/ventilation (B), circulation and bleeding (C), disability and exposure (D,E).[3,10] Patients presenting to an emergency department with a trans-mediastinal injury will often do so in extremis, requiring rapid resuscitative efforts with thoracotomy to identify and treat injuries that are discovered. The uppermost goal in the management of those in extremis is hemorrhage control.[3,9] **Fig. 3** outlines the management strategies for unstable penetrating thoracic injury. **Fig. 4** lists the management for stable penetrating chest trauma and **Fig. 5** describes general management for blunt thoracic trauma.

Specific Injury Patterns and Surgical Techniques

If patients have an identified pneumothorax or hemothorax but are awake with stable hemodynamics, a thoracostomy/chest tube is placed. If the tube drains 1000 to 1500 mL or more, urgent operative intervention is required. If less than a liter drains, the nurse will monitor the drainage and if more than 100 to 200 mL drain on an hourly basis, surgical evaluation is needed.[3,9,20] Injured structures may be repaired primarily or in cases of severe organ damage with persistent bleeding or contamination, structures may be resected. For example, lung injuries may require a wedge resection, lobectomy, or pneumonectomy. Surgeons may perform video-assisted-thorascopic surgery to facilitate any of these procedures.[1]

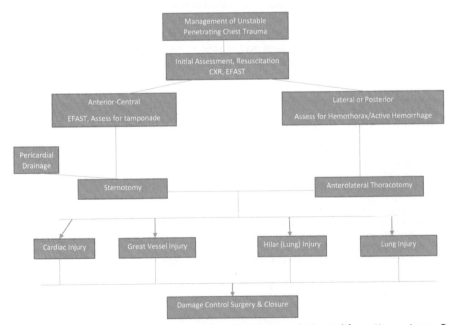

Fig. 3. Management of unstable penetrating chest trauma. (*Adapted from*: Karmy-Jones, R, Namias, N, Coimbra, R, et al. Western Trauma Association critical decisions in trauma: penetrating chest trauma. J Trauma Acute Care Surg 2014; 77(6): 994-1002.)

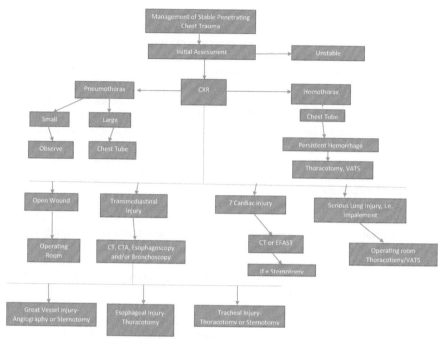

Fig. 4. Management of stable penetrating chest trauma. (*Adapted from*: Karmy-Jones, R, Namias, N, Coimbra, R, et al. Western Trauma Association critical decisions in trauma: penetrating chest trauma. *J Trauma Acute Care Surg* 2014; 77(6): 994-1002.)

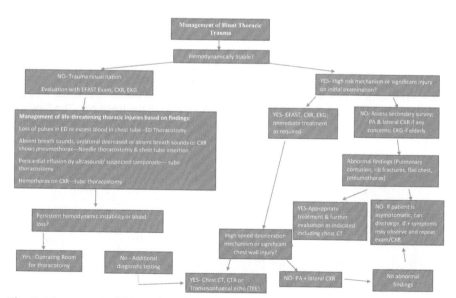

Fig. 5. Managment of blunt thoracic trauma. (*Adapted from*: Whizar-Lugo, V, Sauceda-Gastelum, A, Hernández-Armas, A, et al, (2015). Chest trauma: an overview. J Anesth Crit Care Open Access 2015; 3(1): 00082.)

Surgeons use information on the mechanism, trajectory of penetration, imaging, and amount of chest tube drainage to guide surgical interventions. The surgical incision may be a left or right anterolateral thoracotomy, a bilateral anterolateral thoracotomy, or a median sternotomy (**Fig. 6**).[9] These procedures are frequently performed in the emergency department to treat hemorrhage, to release cardiac tamponade, to cross-clamp the descending thoracic aorta and to fluid-resuscitate. An emergency department thoracotomy (EDT) with aortic cross-clamping allows for occlusion of the aorta to prevent exsanguination. An EDT is indicated for patients with penetrating thoracic injuries who present in extremis with signs of life (**Box 2**). Patients presenting in shock due to hemorrhage should undergo EDT or be taken to the operating room for a potentially life-saving procedure.[1,23,24] The aim of EDT is to restore cardiac output and effective cardiac rhythm and to prevent exsanguination in patients with impending cardiovascular collapse.[23–25]

Blunt injury to the aorta may be managed with blood pressure control and possible surgical intervention to oversew a tear or laceration or to place grafting material, bridging a larger defect. Placement of endovascular stent grafts is the most common intervention for this injury and is known as thoracic endovascular aortic repair.[1,26,27] The Society for Vascular Surgery recommends lower severity injuries such as an intimal tear or hematoma be managed conservatively. Higher grade injuries such as free rupture of the aorta require surgery.[3,28]

Penetrating cardiac injury requires operative control through thoracotomy. The wound may be primarily repaired with suturing with control of bleeding first gained with an occluding finger, vascular clamp, or balloon inflation. Cardiopulmonary bypass may be used to facilitate closure of posterior left ventricular wounds close to coronary arteries.[1]

Blunt cardiac injury management includes supportive care, monitoring of cardiac status and symptom management. Cardiogenic shock is managed with invasive or noninvasive hemodynamic monitoring, and cardioactive medications as needed.[17] Patients with cardiac/pericardial tamponade require an intervention to relieve the tamponade such as pericardiocentesis (**Fig. 7**), or emergent thoracotomy. A pericardial window may also be surgically created to promote continued drainage of fluid.[1,14,17,29] Indications for surgical management after blunt cardiac injury include hemodynamic instability suspicious for cardiac injuries or other vascular injuries.[2,3,17]

Rib fixation surgery for the management of rib fractures is becoming more commonplace. This surgical intervention, performed with various rib fixation systems, may be used when respiratory failure occurs presumably related to the fractures. The Eastern Association for the Surgery of Trauma recommends the use of rib plating to improve

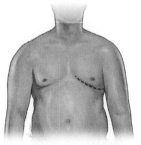
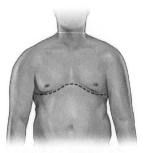
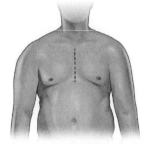

Left anterolateral thoracotomy   Bilateral anterolateral thoracotomy   Midline sternotomy

Fig. 6. Surgical incisions for thoracic trauma.

Box 2
Indications for Emergent Thoracotomy in Chest Trauma

Indications for Emergent Thoracotomy in Chest Trauma

Patient in extremis with unstable vital signs/cardiopulmonary arrest

More than 1000 mL drained via thoracostomy (chest) tube on insertion or within the first one-half hour after placement

Continued drainage of 100 to 200 mL per hour via the chest tube after the initial liter

Refractory hypotension

Large air leak via the chest tube with potential for trachea, bronchus, or esophageal injury

Cardiac/pericardial tamponade

---

outcomes.[30] A recent meta-analysis identified that rib fixation provided benefit for patients with rib fractures in length of stay, mortality, and pneumonia. However, the subgroup older than 60 years had improved outcomes with conservative therapy. Appropriate patient selection is needed when considering interventions.[31] Sternal fractures and other chest wall injuries may require more than conservative management or noninvasive interventions. Surgical interventions such as fixation of ribs as described or open sternal reduction or elevation with fixation may be required.[31]

Additional Management Strategies

Large bore intravenous lines and fluid resuscitation are mainstays of the management of patients with bleeding due to chest trauma. Injuries to the cardiac box or those with a transmediastinal trajectory that may have caused injury to the superior vena cava require central lines placed in the common femoral vein to ensure fluids remain in the intravascular space.[1] Patients may require invasive or noninvasive determinations of fluid requirements once the acute resuscitative period is complete. Judicious fluid administration is needed during this period, especially in the elderly. A central venous

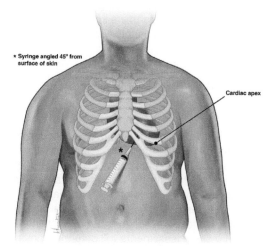

* Syringe angled 45° from surface of skin

Cardiac apex

Fig. 7. Pericardiocentecis for cardiac tamponade. *Adapted from* Whizar-Lugo, V, Sauceda-Gastelum, A, Hernández-Armas, A, et al, (2015). Chest trauma: an overview. J Anesth Crit Care Open Access 2015; 3(1): 00082.

catheter may be used to measure central venous pressure in elderly patients, especially those with pulmonary or cardiac injury.[1] A pulmonary artery catheter may have a role in determining cardiac pressures and fluid volume requirements.

Permissive hypotension may be used in some situations for hemorrhage control to prevent the disruption of adherent clot.[9] Resuscitation may be limited to what is necessary to maintain mentation and urine output and not to achieving a specific blood pressure.[1] In fluid resuscitation in unstable patients, products are administered in a fixed ratio approaching the constitution of whole blood. Some trauma centers use viscoelastic hemostatic assays to determine the proper blood products for resuscitation. Standard coagulation testing may also be used for this purpose.[9]

Damage control surgery and resuscitation are trauma protocols that encourage early blood administration, increasing red cell to plasma transfusion ratios and monitoring for coagulopathy. These strategies are focused on preventing the lethal triad of acidosis, hypothermia, and coagulopathy by limiting the time factor of the first surgery or intervention.[1,16,32] Nursing interventions to warm the patient, continue goal-directed fluid resuscitation, and prevent the lethal triad are key strategies after damage control surgery. With these actions, nurses prepare patients for subsequent reoperation for severe injuries.

When an injury occurs to the chest, significant pain can contribute splinting/guarding, low tidal volumes with pulmonary complications.[2] Pain control is essential in the management of patients who sustain traumatic chest injury, especially those with rib fractures. Effective pain management improves lung mechanics, increases the ability to take a deep breath, helps mobilize secretions, and decreases the likelihood of pulmonary complications.[1-3]

Narcotics are the mainstay of pain management but can cause respiratory depression, oversedation, and delirium. Multimodal pain management with early nonsteroidal anti-inflammatory drugs has shown to reduce narcotic requirements while improving pain scores and increasing vital capacity.[2,33-36] Regional analgesia with thoracic epidural catheters or nerve blocks (thoracic paravertebral, intercostal nerve, or myofascial plane) are beneficial in providing adequate pain relief with a minimal side effect profile.[1,2]

The nursing role is vital to the management of thoracic trauma through interventions and monitoring. Aggressive interventions including pulmonary hygiene, assisting with incentive spirometry and mobilization efforts are important preventive efforts to avoid the development of complications such as follows:

- Atelectasis
- Pneumonia
- Venous thromboembolism
- Empyema
- Wound or other infections

Critical care nurses monitor the drainage and proper function of tubes and drains, especially chest tubes. An apical chest tube will remove air from the thorax as evidenced by bubbling in the underwater seal chamber. A postero-lateral tube will drain blood and fluids. The nurse monitors for the presence of an air leak.

If major vascular injuries require operative or endovascular repair, nurses will perform assessments in the postoperative/postprocedural phase of treatment. Access sites should be monitored for complications. Embolic events and spinal ischemia can develop postprocedure and assessments will determine any acute changes suggestive of a worsening condition.[19] Compartment syndrome of the lower extremities can occur in any of these situations and nurses will assess for this and other complications on a frequent basis (**Box 3**).

Box 3
Signs of Postinjury or Postintervention Vascular Complications

Signs of Postinjury or Postintervention Vascular Complications

Pain out of proportion to event or new onset of pain

Paresthesia of the affected limb

Loss or decrease of motor function

Loss or decrease of sensory function

Tense swelling of extremity

Diminished or absent pulses in extremity

Elevated measured compartment pressures

SUMMARY

Unfortunately, traumatic chest injuries are encountered with frequency in civilian life. Nurses have the knowledge and expertise to significantly improve the identification and management of thoracic injuries from blunt and penetrating forces. In doing so, nurses may affect the high levels of morbidity and mortality seen in this group of patients and improve outcomes.

CLINICS CARE POINTS

- Pain management.
- Monitor for signs/symptoms of hemorrhage.
- When checking for an air leak in a chest/thoracostomy tube, remove suction source to eliminate false-negative pressure. This prevents false tidaling and bubbling in the underwater seal chamber, which may be interpreted incorrectly as an air leak.
- In a patient with an expanding air leak in chest/thoracotomy tube, requiring additional chest tubes, suspect a mediastinal disruption.[3,9,20]
- Monitor for underlying organ injury in patients with rib fractures of the first 3 ribs. These patients need additional diagnostic testing and can deteriorate quickly.[2]
- Stand at the foot of the patient's bed with rib fractures to best visualize paradoxical chest wall movements of flail chest.
- Look for signs of tension pneumothorax with mediastinal shifting by assessing for tracheal will deviation (pushing away from affected lung).

CASE STUDY

A 23-year-old man found on street with multiple GSWs to the chest and abdomen. *Prehospital*: Transferred immediately to trauma center.

Initial assessment:
- Airway: Patent
- Breathing: Spontaneous, diminished breath sounds on right, RR 30, SpO$_2$ RA 89%
- Circulation: HR ST 140, BP 88/60
  - Bilateral 14 guage intravenous lines placed

- Other: 10/10 Pain
- Exposure: Pale. 6 Bullet wounds
  - 2 Right anterior chest
  - 1 Right back
  - 3 Abdomen

Interventions:
- Right chest tube placed for 1500 mL blood
- Emergent right anterolateral thoracotomy at fifth intercostal space
- Bullet went through the inferior-lateral lung, which was stapled. Another bullet transversed the intercostal artery. Hemorrhage controlled with suture repair of the vessel
- Chest and abdomen packed open. Temporary closure of chest skin alone

Moved to Surgical ICU in critical condition
- Ongoing resuscitation, warming, and correction of coagulopathy
- Received: 6 units of blood, 4 L Crystalloid
- Urine output: 800 cc
- BP: 115/74, HR: 106, RR: 23, SpO_2: 100%
- Remained intubated, ventilated, sedated, received continuous narcotic infusion.

Nurses monitored:
- Chest tube function
- Drainage
- Chest wound and dressing
- 5 L Crystalloid, blood, plasma, platelets given during the first 12 h to maintain BP and urine output. Goal was not for a supranormal BP

Resuscitated to:
Resolution of acidosis
Resolution of coagulopathy
Normothermia
Returned to operating room the next day for definitive repairs and wound closure
Patient stabilized over days and was later transferred to a rehabilitation facility
Questions:
What were the indications for the ED Thoracotomy?
What nursing interventions contributed to the positive outcomes in this case?

DECLARATION OF INTERESTS

The author has no commercial or financial conflicts of interest.

REFERENCES

1. Feliciano DV, Dubose JJ. Cardiac, great vessel, and pulmonary injuries. In: Rasmussen TE, editor. *Rich's vascular surgery.* 4th edition. Philadelphia: Elsevier; 2022. p. 171–98.
2. Kim M, Moore JE. Chest trauma: current recommendations for rib fractures & other injuries. Curr Anesthesiol Reports 2020;10(1):61–8.
3. Mert Ü, Andruszkow H, Hildebrand F. Chest trauma. In: Pape H.C., *Textbook of polytrauma management.* 3rd edition. New York: Springer; 2022. p. 161–84.
4. O'Donovan S, van den Heuvel C, Baldock M, et al. Fatal blunt chest trauma: an evaluation of rib fracture patterns and age. Int J Legal Med 2022;136(5):1351–7.
5. El-Menyar A, Latifi R, AbdulRahman H, et al. Age and traumatic chest injury: a 3-year study. Euro J Trauma Emerg Surg 2013;39(4):397–403.

6. Tran J, Haussner W, Shah K. Traumatic pneumothorax. J Emerg Med 2021;2021: 517–28.

7. Edgecombe L, Sigmon DF, Galuska MA, et al. Thoracic trauma. StatPearls. 2022. Available at: https://europepmc.org/article/nbk/nbk534843. Accessed July 22, 2022.

8. Bagaria V, Mathur P, Madan K, et al. Predicting outcomes after blunt chest trauma. Indian J Surg 2021;83(1):113–9.

9. Jogiat Uzair M, Strickland M. Transmediastinal penetrating trauma. Mediastinum 2021;5.

10. American College of Surgeons Committee on Trauma. ATLS student course manual. 10th edition. Chicago: American College of Surgeons; 2018.

11. de Lesquen H, Avaro JP, Gust L, et al. Surgical management for the first 48 hours following blunt chest trauma. Interactive Cardiovasc Thorac Surg 2015;20(3): 399–408.

12. Mahmood I, El-Menyar A, Younis B, et al. Clinical significance and prognostic implications of quantifying pulmonary contusion volume in patients with blunt chest trauma. Med Sci Monitor: Internatl Med J of Experiment & Clin Res 2017;23:3641.

13. El Mestoui Z, Jalalzadeh H, Giannakopoulos GF, et al. Incidence and etiology of mortality in polytrauma patients. Eur J Emerg Med 2017;24(1):49–54.

14. Selvakumar S, Newsome K, Nguyen T, et al. The role of pericardial window techniques in the management of penetrating cardiac injuries in the hemodynamically stable patient. J Surg Res 2022;276:120–35.

15. Dahal R, Acharya Y, Tyroch AH, et al. Blunt thoracic aortic injury & contemporary management strategy. Angiology 2022;73(6):497–507.

16. Spahn DR, Bouillon B, Cerny V, et al. The European guideline on management of bleeding and coagulopathy following trauma. Crit Care 2019;23(1):1–74.

17. Shoar S, Hosseini FS, Naderan M, et al. Cardiac injury following blunt chest trauma. Internatl J Burns & Trauma 2021;11(2):80.

18. Gao JM, Li H, Wei GB, et al. Blunt cardiac injury: a single-center 15-year experience. Am Surg 2020;86(4):354–61.

19. Monga A, Patil SB, Cherian M, et al. Thoracic trauma: aortic injuries. Semin Intervent Radiol 2021;38:1–38.

20. Clemente AG, Lima JH, Yazbek BO, et al. Esophageal trauma. In: Nasr A, editor. *The trauma golden hour.* New York: Springer; 2020. p. 101–5.

21. Keng LT, Yang HC. Use of eFAST in patients with injury to the thorax or abdomen. N Engl J Med 2022;386(20):1963–4.

22. Stojanovska J, Koweek LMH, Chung JH, et al. ACR appropriateness criteria® blunt chest trauma-cardiac injury. J American Coll Radiol 2020;17(11):S380–90.

23. Liu A, Nguyen J, Ehrlich H, et al. Emergency resuscitative thoracotomy for civilian thoracic trauma in the field and emergency department settings: a systematic review. J Surg Res 2022;273:44–55.

24. Panossian VS, Nederpelt CJ, El Hechi MW, et al. Emergency resuscitative thoracotomy. J Surg Res 2020;255:486–94.

25. Refaely Y, Koyfman L, Friger M, et al. Clinical outcome of urgent thoracotomy in patients with penetrating & blunt chest trauma. Thorac Cardiovasc Surg 2018; 66(8):686–92.

26. Scalea TM, Feliciano DV, DuBose JJ, et al. Blunt thoracic aortic injury: endovascular repair is now the standard. J Am Coll Surg 2019;228(4):605–10.

27. Hundersmarck D, van der Vliet QM, Winterink LM, et al. Blunt thoracic aortic injury and TEVAR. Eur J Trauma Emerg Surg 2020;2020:1–13.

28. DuBose JJ, Leake SS, Brenner M, et al. Contemporary management and outcomes of blunt thoracic aortic injury: a multicenter retrospective study. J Trauma Acute Care Surg 2015;78(2):360–9.

29. Alerhand S, Adrian RJ, Long B, et al. Pericardial tamponade: a comprehensive review. Am J Emerg Med 2022;2022:159–74.

30. Kasotakis G, Hasenboehler EA, Streib EW, et al. Operative fixation of rib fractures after blunt trauma: guideline from EAST. J Trauma Acute Care Surg 2017;82(3): 618–26.

31. Sawyer E, Wullschleger M, Muller N, et al. Surgical rib fixation of multiple rib fractures and flail chest: a systematic review. J Surg Res 2022;276:221–34.

32. Roberts DJ, Ball CG, Feliciano DV, et al. History of the innovation of damage control for management of trauma patients. Ann Surg 2017;265(5):1034–44.

33. Brasel KJ, Moore EE, Albrecht RA, et al. Western trauma association critical decisions in trauma: management of rib fractures. J Trauma Acute Care Surg 2017; 82(1):200–3.

34. Galvagno SM, Smith CE, Varon AJ. Pain management for blunt thoracic trauma: guideline from the eastern association for the surgery of trauma and trauma anesthesiology society. J Trauma Acute Care Surg 2016;81(5):936–51.

35. Karmy-Jones R, Namias N, Coimbra R, et al. Western Trauma Association: penetrating chest trauma. J Trauma Acute Care Surg 2014;77(6):994–1002 (Reference for Figs. 4 & 5).

36. Whizar-Lugo V, Sauceda-Gastelum A, Hernández-Armas A, et al. Chest trauma: an overview. J Anesth Crit Care Open Access 2015;3(1):82 (Reference for Fig. 7).

Ethical Challenges in the Care of the Trauma Patient

Maureen Frances McLaughlin, MS, RN, ACNS-BC, CPAN, CAPA

KEYWORDS

- Nursing care • Health care • Beneficence • Pulseless electrical activity
- Electrocardiogram • Emergency department • Cardiopulmonary resuscitation
- Ethical principles

Integral to the nursing care of patients is adherence to an ingrained, long-taught code of nursing ethics. However, the provision of care to the emergent trauma patient may not always align with these ethical principles due to the emergent nature of the traumatic event that by its very suddenness precludes autonomous advanced care planning, family discussions, or other contemplative processes that are possible with planned surgery and/or procedures. Equally unique in the care of the patient with trauma is that the provision of care is nonrelationship based because the patient typically is not known to the care team or to the facility. Ethical challenges develop because the trauma team frequently does not know the wishes and desires of the patient and must make decisions rapidly based on their expert clinical judgment.

Ethical principles are guidelines, rules, or standards for action that are designed to guide decision-making based on what is good for humans.[1] Ethical principles frequently used and cited in nursing practice include beneficence, nonmaleficence, autonomy, justice, fidelity, and veracity.

The principle of beneficence is the duty to do good. Beneficence is the cornerstone of the provision of health care and may be interpreted as the "duty to maximize benefits and reduce harm to patients."[2] The ethical principle of nonmaleficence simply stated is the obligation to do no harm. Although appearing to interrelate, there are clinical scenarios in which these principles may actually be in conflict with each other.

The ethical principle of justice addresses just and fair allocation of health-care resources and nursing care to patients.

Autonomy is the ethical principle that states individuals ought to be able to make their own decisions, often described as self-determination.

The ethical principle of veracity is simply stated as the obligation to tell the truth. Finally, the ethical principle of fidelity is the duty to remain faithful to one's commitments, implicit in a patient–nurse relationship.

Department of Anesthesiology, Lahey Hospital and Medical Center, 41 Mall Road, Burlington, MA 01805, USA
E-mail address: maureen.f.mclaughlin@lahey.org

Crit Care Nurs Clin N Am 35 (2023) 145–149
https://doi.org/10.1016/j.cnc.2023.02.006
ccnursing.theclinics.com

CASE STUDY

An 89-year-old female patient brought in by ambulance from a skilled nursing facility where she had been recovering following a fall with injuries. The patient had been found unresponsive and pulseless in her room; resuscitation was initiated by facility, and 911 was called. Return of spontaneous circulation (ROSC) was achieved following chest compressions and epinephrine, which was administered for a rhythm determined to be pulseless electrical activity. During transport to the nearest facility, pulses were lost again and cardiopulmonary resuscitation (CPR) resumed; ROSC again achieved. The patient was intubated by emergency medical services (EMS) during transport. On admission to the emergency department (ED), the staff identified that the patient had a medical order for life sustaining treatment (MOLST), which stated do-not-resuscitate (DNR)/do-not-intubate (DNI). Although the providers attempted to reach the patient's family by phone, on-going resuscitation was continued including rainbow laboratory testing, electrocardiogram (EKG), and vasopressor therapy for the treatment of hypotension. An epinephrine infusion was also initiated. The ED attending was able to contact the patient's son who resided a distance away and was not able to come to the facility. The son requested that the team continue all efforts to save his mother. The patient was transferred to the intensive care unit (ICU) for further care and management. An arterial and a central line were placed. Full ventilatory support was provided. A neurologic examination revealed fixed and dilated pupils; no spontaneous movement was noted during a pause in sedation. The following morning, the ICU contacted the son and provided a detailed summary of their clinical findings including radiographic evidence of cerebral anoxia, 3 rib fractures, likely aspiration pneumonia, and EKG changes indicative of ischemia. The ICU team stressed the very poor prognosis and encouraged the son to consider the cessation of further heroic measures. It remained unclear whether the son was aware of the MOLST form and/or his mother's directives for end-of-life care. The son wished to confer with other family members and did not make a decision at that time. The patient experienced worsening hemodynamic instability and additional vasopressors were initiated. The team contacted the son again and stressed that it was unlikely that his mother would survive much longer. He agreed to transition his mother to DNR and halt any further escalation in pharmacologic management but not comfort measures only (CMO). The patient passed later that morning.

DISCUSSION

Acting on the premise of the patient self-determination act, this patient had expressed her wish that no life-sustaining measures be used to prolong her life.[1,3] This information was known to the ED staff; it is unclear if it was known to the staff at the skilled nursing facility. Despite that knowledge, the ED provider contacted the patient's next of kin (NOK) who desired that all life-sustaining measures be attempted.

There are several ethical issues in this case study. The ethical principle of autonomy was not supported by the ED provider; despite the advanced directive present, the staff deferred the decision-making to her NOK. The ethical principles of beneficence and nonmaleficence are in conflict as well. Efforts to do good by continuing life-sustaining measures was in juxtaposition to do no harm because life-sustaining measures were in fact contradictory to the patient's previously stated wishes. Fidelity is perhaps another ethical principle challenged in this case study. The nursing encounter, while brief and without a prior nurse–patient relationship, as in many trauma situations, was in conflict with the patient's stated wishes of DNR/DNI.

CASE STUDY

A 21-year-old male patient was transported by Med Flight to a Level 1 trauma center following a motorcycle accident in which he was thrown approximately 50 feet off his bike. He was not wearing a helmet. Posturing was noted by the med flight team at the scene, and hypertonic saline was administered. On arrival in the ED, the patient was emergently intubated and massive transfusion protocol was initiated due to hemodynamic instability. Imaging revealed extensive injuries including grade IV liver laceration, multiple fractures including ribs, clavicles and bilateral lower extremities, burst fractures in the cervical spine and perhaps most concerning, subarachnoid hemorrhage with a midline shift. Given the emergent nature of his injuries, the patient underwent an embolization in Interventional Radiology for stabilization of the liver injury and emergency craniectomy to decompress the worsening intracranial pressure. The patient was of course unable to consent to these procedures; presumed consent was used given the patient's age and urgent nature of his injuries. The area police department was attempting to both accurately identify the patient and locate NOK.

During the course of the following days, the ICU team further managed the extensive injuries the young man sustained. Family had been located and included mother with whom the patient resided; father, previously divorced from the mother and estranged from the family; and 2 younger siblings. Not surprisingly given his young age, no advanced directive was reported to exist.

On hospital day 5, a family meeting was convened to update the family on the progress of treatment and discuss future care. Imaging had revealed extensive anoxic areas in the brain; the patient was unresponsive without evidence of movement without pharmacologic sedation. In addition, the family was informed that the cervical spine injuries would likely result in permanent paralysis even if surgical stabilization were to take place. A tracheostomy and peg tube placement would need to occur in the near future if the family wished to pursue on-going aggressive treatment. A neurologist who participated in the family meeting stated that in his expert opinion the patient had suffered an irreversible brain injury and would likely persist in a chronic vegetative state if he survived.

The family was expectedly devastated by the team summary. The patient's mother responded that her son would never wish to live in such a disabled state. The patient's father, however, stated that it was premature to have this type of discussion and wanted to continue aggressive care and treatment. Because the patient could not speak for himself and was no longer a juvenile, the social worker involved in the case stated that the family needed to pursue guardianship to determine who had decision-making authority.

During the course of the following week, the team noted increasing conflict between the patient's parents. Both wished to be the patient's guardian and legal consultation was required. The ICU team continued to aggressively manage the patient worsening clinical status, which now included pneumonia, seizures, rising intracranial pressure and concerns for brain stem herniation. On hospital day 12, the nurse caring for the patient noted bilateral fixed and dilated pupils; a stat CT scan was performed. During the course of the next 12 hours, brain death was determined by neurologic criteria. The family was able to agree together to a DNR status and to pursue organ donation with the assistance of the local organ bank.

DISCUSSION

Ethical principles challenged in this case study include beneficence, nonmaleficence, autonomy, and perhaps fidelity.[1,3] The young man not surprisingly had not discussed end of life issues with his parents and had not completed a health-care proxy. His actual wishes were unknown and given the critical nature of his injuries, he was unable to make health-care decisions autonomously for himself. Family dynamics did not align with clear decision-making given the conflicting opinions of the parents. The health-care team wished to provide the best care for the patient but in so doing was prolonging the life of a young man with a devastating traumatic brain injury without hope for a meaningful recovery: beneficence and nonmaleficence in opposition perhaps. The nursing staff remained faithful to both the patient and the family and continued to provide expert compassionate care in the management of the patient's extensive injuries without judgment or prejudice because the family members struggled to make health-care decisions for their son.

CASE STUDY

Two victims, a man and a woman, both suffering from serious gunshot injuries, are brought to the same trauma center amid extensive police and media coverage. The female patient suffered multiple injuries reportedly from her former husband against whom the court had recently approved a restraining order on behalf of this patient. Her injuries included multiple stab wounds to the torso, attempted strangulation, and a gunshot wound to the head. Per police at the scene, the male victim was the woman's former husband who had reportedly violated the restraining order and assaulted his former wife. Police had responded to a 911 call placed from the residence and shots were fired; the second victim per EMS suffered a gunshot wounds to the abdomen and lower extremity.

Both victims were transported to the closest trauma center. The female patient arrived intubated, unresponsive, and hemodynamically unstable; massive transfusion protocol was initiated. She became pulseless at one point but ROSC was achieved following 10 minutes of resuscitation. Injuries identified by the trauma team included grade III liver laceration, multiple superficial stab wounds, and concerns for traumatic brain injury due to the gunshot wound. Her Glasgow Coma Scale was assessed at 3T. The stab wounds were quickly sutured in the emergency room and the patient was brought emergently to the operating room for a craniotomy.

The second patient arrived awake and combative; he was electively intubated to better manage the primary and secondary survey. After imaging and laboratory work were completed, he was brought emergently to the operating room (OR) for an exploratory laparotomy and wound exploration of his lower extremity.

Both patients were transported to the surgical intensive care unit (SICU) following surgery; their names remained the assigned trauma nomenclature used for as yet unidentified trauma victims. The SICU footprint was large and the patients were separated into 2 separate pods. Resources were mobilized to address media coverage, family support and the on-going police investigation.

During the course of the following 2 days, the female patient's condition worsened. Her neurologic examination remained poor: pupils nonreactive and no spontaneous movement. Her NOK was determined to be her brother. Fortunately, a health-care proxy form was located listing the brother as the proxy. Social work and palliative care were consulted.

The male patient was extubated on postoperative day 1. His injuries were determined to be nonlife threatening and he was transferred to an inpatient unit with a police detail.

The media continued to barrage the SICU with phone calls seeking information on both patients, proving to be a large distraction and stressor for the nursing staff.

On hospital day number 10, the female patient was transitioned to CMO and passed peacefully without ever regaining consciousness. On hospital day number 6, the male patient was transferred to a rehabilitation facility. Criminal charges had been brought against him for the reported attack on his former wife.

DISCUSSION

This case study while tragic is not uncommon; ICUs must care for both the victim and at times the assailant.[1,3] The ethical principle of justice predominates in this case study. The critical care nurses were obligated to provide the same competent, expert, compassionate care to both the female and male patients regardless of the criminal and tragic nature of the events. The ethical principle of fidelity is also relevant to this case study. The nurses knew to keep all patient information confidential and not discuss events with anyone not directly involved with the patient's care, including family and friends or even other staff nurses. The organization ensured that a separate team of nurses cared for each patient while they were in the SICU to ease some of the care burden.

SUMMARY

A patient with trauma presents a unique and/or complex challenge to the ethical foundation that guides nursing care. Patients with trauma, by the very nature of the suddenness of their injury, are unable to predetermine or express their wishes in the event of a catastrophic injury. The providers who care for patients with trauma do not have an established patient relationship to aid them in decision-making based on what they think the patient would wish or based on past conversations. Yet, all who care for a patient with trauma provide expert care and use well-defined ethical principles to direct their professional responsibility to these patients.

CLINICS CARE POINTS

- Nurses should be familiar with ethical principles.
- Healthcare providers must respect patient's autonomy in their decision-making.
- In emergency situations where an informed consent is not achievable, presumed consent may be used to save a patient's life.

REFERENCES

1. Grace PJ, editor. Nursing ethics and professional responsibility. Third ed. Burlington, MA: Jones & Bartlett Learning; 2018.
2. Scarlet S. Caring for the wounded: ethics of trauma surgery. AMA J Ethics 2018; 20(5):421–4.
3. Angelos S. How should trauma patients informed consent or refusal be regarded in a trauma bay or other emergency settings? AMA J Ethics 2018;20(5):425–30.

Geriatric Trauma and Frailty
Improving Outcomes Through Multidisciplinary Care

Whitney Villegas, DNP, APRN, AGACNP-BC[a,b,*]

KEYWORDS

- Trauma • Geriatric • Elderly • Frail • Frailty

KEY POINTS

- Geriatric patients have decreased ability to handle the stress of traumatic injuries, and those with frailty are at the highest risk of poor outcomes in trauma.
- Multi-disciplinary care can improve outcomes in frail geriatric trauma patients, including mortality, morbidity, length of stay, and discharge disposition.
- The bedside critical care nurse is a vital member of the multi-disciplinary team in improving geriatric trauma outcomes.

INTRODUCTION

The geriatric population in the United States is increasing with subsequent increasing rates of geriatric trauma.[1] According to the 2016 National Trauma Data Bank, greater than 30% of patients with trauma are aged older than 65 years,[2] and this number is expected to increase to 40% by the year 2050.[3] The most common mechanism of injury for this age group is falls, accounting for 76% of injuries; motor vehicle crashes account for approximately 11.5% of injuries.[2] There is no consistent understanding of which age should be considered geriatric in trauma. Age 65 is typically considered geriatric due to Medicare rules, and many trauma organizations (such as the Eastern Association of Surgical Trauma) use this age in their care guidelines to define the geriatric population.[4] However, trauma data has shown increased mortality and morbidity for the top 3 mechanisms starting at 57 years of age.[2]

COMPLEXITY OF GERIATRIC TRAUMA

Caring for patients with geriatric trauma is extremely complex because they have decreased ability to handle the physical stress of injuries due to age-related changes, and the vast majority has chronic medical problems.[5] As a result, these patients have

[a] Texas Tech University, Lubbock, TX, USA; [b] JPS Health Network, 1500 South Main Street, Fort Worth, TX 76104, USA
* 1500 South Main Street, Fort Worth, TX 76104.
E-mail addresses: Whitney.villegas@ttuhsc.edu; wvillega@jpshealth.org

Crit Care Nurs Clin N Am 35 (2023) 151–160
https://doi.org/10.1016/j.cnc.2023.02.007
0899-5885/23/© 2023 Elsevier Inc. All rights reserved.
ccnursing.theclinics.com

worse outcomes in terms of survival and disability compared with younger patients with trauma.[1,3,5] Traumatic brain injuries are major cause of death in patients with geriatric trauma, and the overall 1-year mortality for hip fractures is 21.2%.[6] Common complications in geriatric trauma are pneumonia, urinary tract infections, deep vein thrombosis/thrombophlebitis, acute kidney injury, respiratory failure, and decubitus ulcers.[2] All hospitalized elderly patients are at risk for developing delirium, a sudden onset of confusion and dysfunction of thought. Delirium leads to longer hospital stays, higher mortality, and decreased likelihood to discharge home.[3]

There is a wide range of physical functioning in the elderly population; one 70-year-old patient may play tennis 3 times per week, whereas another patient of the same age may struggle to ambulate.[7] Every human body undergoes a gradual deterioration over time in a process called senescence, which can increase the risk of traumatic events (Fig. 1). An overall reduction in muscle mass and strength can lead to falls, and a decline in processing speeds can affect response times while driving.[8] Spinal rigidity can also make older patients more susceptible to injuries of the cervical spine.[6] The body's ability to maintain homeostasis during times of physiologic stress also significantly declines over time. In elderly trauma patients, the inability to mount a stress response and use of beta blockers can mask the presence of hemorrhage.[6] Some trauma research has indicated that a systolic blood pressure less than 110 in a trauma patient aged older than 65 years should be considered hypotensive during the initial trauma evaluation.[9] Lack of adequate compensatory mechanisms can also lead to significant hemodynamic instability.

Chronic medical conditions significantly contribute to the complexity of caring for patients with geriatric trauma. Patients with osteoporosis can sustain fractures and dislocations even with minor trauma, and neurocognitive impairments such as dementia can make it challenging to detect injuries.[6] Wound healing can be adversely

Cardiovascular	Pulmonary
• Decreased cardiac output, myocardial compliance • Decrease SA node cells: Increased risk of dysrhythmias • Increased vagal tone: Decreased basal heart rate	• Decreased elastic recoil: Increased lung compliance • Loss of respiratory muscle mass: More rapid breathing and reduced cough ability • Increased ventilation/perfusion mismatch • Decreased mucus production; reduced cough

Senescence

Hepatorenal	Skin and Musculoskeletal
• Decreased renal mass and renal blood flow with decline in GFR • Reduced ability to metabolize drugs	• Atrophy and denervation of sensory and motor systems • Reduced skin collagen and elastin • Reduced overall muscle mass and strength

Fig. 1. Age-related physiologic changes.[8] *Adapted from* Yang R, Wolfson M, Lewis MC. Unique aspects of the elderly surgical population: An anesthesiologist's perspective. Geriatr Orthop Surg Rehabil 2011,2(2),56-64. doi:10.1177/21514585103946064.

affected by diabetes and poor blood flow (such as in peripheral artery disease). Although not the primary reason for admission, chronic illnesses must continue to be managed while the patient is hospitalized for trauma, which may include blood pressure control, preventing hyperglycemia and hypoglycemia, administering home oxygen, and restarting necessary home medications.

A major cause of falls in the elderly is polypharmacy.[6] The American Geriatrics Society has created the Beers Criteria to outline inappropriate medications for geriatric patients.[10] Commonly used medications that can alter mentation and contribute to falls include opioids, anticholinergics (such as diphenhydramine and promethazine), benzodiazepines (lorazepam, alprazolam, and clonazepam), some antidepressants, and muscle relaxants. Gabapentin and pregabalin should also be used cautiously in combination with opioids. Orthostatic hypotension caused by blood pressure medications can also lead to falls and traumatic injuries.[10] Certain medications can cause significant problems after trauma is sustained, and the most dangerous are "blood thinning" medications, such as warfarin, novel oral anticoagulants, and antiplatelet agents.[10] Patients who take these medications can have life-threatening bleeding even with seemingly minor trauma, either from exsanguination or from intracranial hemorrhage.

Frailty

A more accurate predictor than age of outcomes in trauma is the presence of frailty.[6] Frailty is a clinical syndrome resulting from the progressive loss of physiologic reserves across multiple body systems that makes patients more vulnerable during acute events of stress.[6,7] Frail patients typically have a combination of poor nutrition, decreased strength and function, and chronic medical conditions.[7] Patients with frailty are more likely to sustain a traumatic event and multiple studies have shown that patients with frail trauma have worse outcomes compared with those who are not frail. Patients with frail trauma have increased mortality, morbidity, in-hospital and postoperative complications, length of stay (LOS), and readmission rates, as well as adverse discharge disposition.[11–14] As a result, the frail geriatric trauma population significantly contributes to health-care costs due to increased lengths of stay, complications, and readmission rates.[13]

Early identification of frailty is important to develop strategies to improve the patient's health status and prevent further deterioration. Some programs use computed tomography for objective frailty screening by evaluating for decreased muscle mass and quality[15] but this method has not been considered feasible or cost-effective by most programs. Frailty is commonly diagnosed by one of the many screening tools, which can be administered by the provider or bedside nurse. There is no consensus on which tool can best identify frailty but certain tools are more appropriate for use in the emergency department and inpatient setting. Many tools require extended time to administer and direct observation of the patient's gait, which is often not possible in patients with geriatric trauma.[15] In the emergency department, a simple tool with shorter administration time is the most feasible.[16] The 15-item Trauma Specific Frailty Index was specifically developed for the trauma population and has shown to be effective in predicting frailty and outcomes.[7] Especially useful in the emergency department, the Clinical Frailty Score assigns patients a score from 1 (very fit) to 9 (terminally ill) (**Fig. 2**).[17] A newer scale, The Frailty Screening Questionnaire (FSQ), consists of 5 self-reported questions on the domains of unintentional weight loss, weakness, exhaustion, slowness, and inactivity (**Table 1**). The FSQ has a great potential for widespread use in trauma because it is specific and reliable for identifying frailty, can

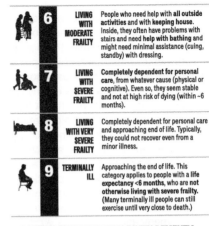

CLINICAL FRAILTY SCALE

1	**VERY FIT**	People who are robust, active, energetic and motivated. They tend to exercise regularly and are among the fittest for their age.
2	**FIT**	People who have **no active disease symptoms** but are less fit than category 1. Often, they exercise or are very **active occasionally**, e.g., seasonally.
3	**MANAGING WELL**	People whose **medical problems are well controlled**, even if occasionally symptomatic, but often are **not regularly active** beyond routine walking.
4	**LIVING WITH VERY MILD FRAILTY**	Previously "vulnerable," this category marks early transition from complete independence. While **not dependent** on others for daily help, often **symptoms limit activities.** A common complaint is being "slowed up" and/or being tired during the day.
5	**LIVING WITH MILD FRAILTY**	People who often have **more evident slowing**, and need help with **high order instrumental activities of daily living** (finances, transportation, heavy housework). Typically, mild frailty progressively impairs shopping and walking outside alone, meal preparation, medications and begins to restrict light housework.
6	**LIVING WITH MODERATE FRAILTY**	People who need help with **all outside activities** and with **keeping house.** Inside, they often have problems with stairs and need **help with bathing** and might need minimal assistance (cuing, standby) with dressing.
7	**LIVING WITH SEVERE FRAILTY**	**Completely dependent for personal care**, from whatever cause (physical or cognitive). Even so, they seem stable and not at high risk of dying (within ~6 months).
8	**LIVING WITH VERY SEVERE FRAILTY**	Completely dependent for personal care and approaching end of life. Typically, they could not recover even from a minor illness.
9	**TERMINALLY ILL**	Approaching the end of life. This category applies to people with a **life expectancy <6 months**, who are **not** otherwise living with severe frailty. (Many terminally ill people can still exercise until very close to death.)

SCORING FRAILTY IN PEOPLE WITH DEMENTIA

The degree of frailty generally corresponds to the degree of dementia. Common **symptoms** in **mild dementia** include forgetting the details of a recent event, though still remembering the event itself, repeating the same question/story and social withdrawal.

In **moderate dementia**, recent memory is very impaired, even though they seemingly can remember their past life events well. They can do personal care with prompting.

In **severe dementia**, they cannot do personal care without help.

In **very severe dementia** they are often bedfast. Many are virtually mute.

DALHOUSIE UNIVERSITY
www.geriatricmedicineresearch.ca

Clinical Frailty Scale ©2005–2020 Rockwood, Version 2.0 (EN). All rights reserved. For permission: www.geriatricmedicineresearch.ca Rockwood K et al. A global clinical measure of fitness and frailty in elderly people. CMAJ 2005;173:489–495.

Fig. 2. Rockwood clinical frailty scale. Clinical Frailty Scale. From: https://www.dal.ca/sites/gmr/our-tools/clinical-frailty-scale.html.

be performed quickly with minimal training, and can be obtained from the caregiver for patients who are unable to complete the interview.[18–20]

Geriatric Trauma Care Considerations

On arrival to the emergency department, the geriatric trauma patient should be carefully and thoroughly evaluated. Obtaining an accurate medical/surgical history with

Table 1
Frailty screening questionnaire

Domain	Question	Score
Weight loss	"Have you lost more than 10 pounds in the last year without trying?"	Yes = 1 No = 0
Weakness	"Can you lift or carrying items that are 10 lbs without difficulty?"	Yes = 0 No = 1
Exhaustion	"Do you feel everything takes effort?"	Yes = 1 No = 0
Inactivity	"Do you spend <3 h each week on leisure activities?"	Yes = 1 No = 0
Slowness	"Are you able to walk 250 yards?" (Independently or with assistive device)	Yes = 0 No = 1
		Total = 0 to 5

Total score of 0-1 = non-frail; 2-3 = pre-frail (intermediate frail); 4-5 = frail.
Adapted with permission from Zhang Y, Zhang Y, Li Y, et al. Reliability and validity of the self-reported frailty screening questionnaire in older adults. Ther Adv Chronic Dis 2020;11,1-8. https://doi.org/10.1177/20406223209042.

medication list (especially blood thinners) is essential to develop a comprehensive plan of care and identify increased risk for potential complications. Psychosocial assessment can identify factors contributing to the traumatic event and risks for subsequent trauma or complications. It is important to assess the patient's living situation, what support is available to the patient, and financial factors that may affect compliance to treatment. Elder abuse and/or neglect should also be considered.[6] Given the increased risk of mortality and complications, patients with geriatric trauma should be asked about any preexisting advanced directives soon after arrival to the hospital; if the patient does not have advanced directives, the assessment of code status should be performed. To decrease the hospital LOS and ensure a safe disposition, discharge planning should start on the day of admission.

Pain Management

Pain control is a primary goal in trauma because it improves the patient's overall comfort and facilitates compliance with respiratory treatments, ambulation, and therapies. However, the management of pain can be difficult in elderly patients due to reduced metabolism of medications or chronic pain.[6] Additionally, medications commonly used for acute pain are on the Beers Criteria, including skeletal muscle relaxants, Non-steroidal anti-inflammatory drugs (NSAIDs), opioids, and gabapentin.[10] Both overtreatment and undertreatment of pain can lead to delirium.[6]

For acute pain management, the risks and benefits of each medication must be weighed carefully for each patient. Acetaminophen is a mainstay of treatment due to few side effects, whereas medications with risk of altering mental status should be started at low doses with careful monitoring.[6] Opioids should be used at the lowest effective dosage and used only for a short duration. Ketamine has been used in patients with geriatric trauma to reduce the requirement of opioids but can have psychogenic side effects such as hallucinations. NSAIDs can be effective in reducing pain in trauma but should be used with caution in patients with poor renal function or risk of gastrointestinal bleeding.[6]

Regional anesthesia and ultrasound-guided nerve blocks have become more commonly used to provide pain relief without the side effects of systemic medications.[6] Available to treat multiple types of traumatic injuries, these blocks may be performed as a single injection or through a pump and catheter that are left in place for several days. Nerve blocks are particularly helpful for patients with rib fractures, where coughing and deep breathing is painful but necessary for recovery. Patients with extremity fractures frequently receive blocks to help with postoperative pain.

Prevention of Complications

Due to increased risk of poor outcomes in patients with geriatric trauma (especially those with frailty), care plans are largely focused on improving health status and preventing complications. Patients who need surgery should undergo prompt preoperative workup (unless the surgery is emergent), which often includes standard laboratories (complete blood count, metabolic panel/electrolytes, INR, or coagulation panel), assessment of fluid status through base deficit or lactic acid, and baseline electrocardiogram. Additional workup may be performed per hospital policy or for specific patient needs; for example, a patient with known cardiac disease may require an echocardiogram or cardiac enzymes before surgery. Patients with geriatric trauma must also be medically optimized before surgery to reduce the risk of intraoperative complications. Interventions may include the correction of coagulopathies or reversal of anticoagulants, fluid resuscitation, blood transfusion, replacement of electrolytes, and blood pressure and glucose control. Timing of surgery is important, ideally within

24 hours after hospital admission. In hip fracture patients, delays in operative timing have been associated with increased mortality and complications such as pneumonia, pulmonary embolism, and myocardial infarction.[21]

Management of comorbidities is widely recognized as an essential element in the care of patients with geriatric trauma to prevent complications. Home medications should be carefully reviewed and resumed when appropriate. For patients on blood thinners that have been held or reversed after trauma, careful risk/benefit evaluation should be performed before restarting. Malnutrition negatively affects recovery in patients with geriatric trauma and should be recognized promptly on admission. Hip fracture patients with malnutrition have shown to have an increased risk of mortality and postoperative complications.[22,23] To optimize nutrition, high-protein and energy supplements can increase weight and muscle mass and reduce morbidity.[24]

Restoration of function is a primary goal for multidisciplinary care in elderly patients with trauma because decreased activities of daily living (ADLs) increase the risk of mortality up to 1-year after injury.[22] Early mobilization after injury has shown to improve functionality, prevent delirium, and reduce deconditioning while inpatient.[3,25–30] Many patients and family members require specialized training in fall prevention before discharge.[3,22,25] Early consultation to social work/case management can facilitate discharge planning for safe disposition to prevent readmissions.[3,25,28–32]

Multidisciplinary Care for Trauma Frailty

In their current guidelines for the care of the geriatric patient, the American College of Surgeons (ACS) recommends using interdisciplinary care for vulnerable patients to address their complex needs.[26,27] The components of multidisciplinary care and roles of each discipline are outlined in **Table 2**. The ACS suggests consultations to a provider with geriatric expertise, pharmacy, nutrition, physical and occupational therapies, and social work.[27] Other consultations may also be appropriate, such to speech language pathology (SLP) for patients with difficulty swallowing and palliative care for those who meet criteria based on comorbidities and prognosis.[27] The most vulnerable patients in trauma are those with frailty; therefore, multidisciplinary care is appropriate for these patients.

Consistent with the ACS recommendations, multidisciplinary care has been used in many trauma and hip fracture programs to improve outcomes. Multidisciplinary care has shown to decrease in-hospital mortality and mortality 1 year after discharge,[22,25,29] reduce LOS,[22,25,28,31] and decrease complications, such as pneumonia and urinary tract infections.[28] Studies have also shown increased mobility and ADLs.[29,30] Discharge disposition, an alternative indicator of functionality, has also improved after the implementation of multidisciplinary care[25,30]; for example, more patients who lived independently prior their trauma were able to discharge back home. Specific to frailty in geriatric trauma, the use of multidisciplinary care has resulted in decreased delirium, LOS, loss of independence, and 30-day readmission rates.[3,31] Although multidisciplinary care increases the number of consultations, the reduction in complications, LOS, and readmissions can offset these costs and lead to overall value of care.[25,30,32]

Critical Care Nurse Role in Frailty and Geriatric Trauma

Critical care nurses are vital team members in the care of the patient with frail geriatric trauma and are well positioned to affect outcomes through continuous hands-on interaction (**Box 1**). As the primary caregivers during hospitalization, nurses assist mobilization and ADLs while encouraging participation in specialized therapies. They are also critical for the management of pain through frequent assessment and

Table 2
The roles of multidisciplinary team members in geriatric trauma and frailty

Team Member	Role
Geriatrician/provider with geriatric expertise	• Management of comorbidities and reduction of high-risk or inappropriate medications[25,28,30,34] • Osteoporosis screening and management[22,30] • Advanced planning and determining goals of care[35]
Clinical Pharmacist	• Medication evaluation • Recommendations to reduce inappropriate medications[27,28]
Dietician	• Nutritional assessment/malnutrition screening and recommendations[27,28]
Physical and Occupational Therapist	• Early mobilization[25–30,33] • Teaching and training for fall prevention and mobility[22,25]
Speech Language Pathology	• Swallow assessment for patients at high risk for problems[26,27]
Social Work/Case Management	• Psychosocial assessment • Early discharge planning[25,28–30,32]
Palliative Care	• Determining goals of care • Facilitate comfort care and/or hospice in patients who meets criteria[27,28]

administration of pharmacologic and nonpharmacologic measures. Risks and symptoms of complications, such as fever or possible aspiration, are often identified and reported by the bedside nurse.

Bedside nurses play an important role in the prevention of delirium in this high-risk population. Nonpharmacologic bedside interventions are most effective in preventing

Box 1
Nursing role in geriatric trauma and frailty

Monitor and Prevent Complications
• Aspiration precautions (sit upright if able)
• Mobilization
• Delirium prevention interventions
• Monitor and report changes in vital signs, mental status, and so forth
• Reduce inappropriate medications

Pain control and Comfort
• Nonpharmacologic pain interventions (repositioning, distraction, music, and so forth)
• Pain medications with follow-up assessment
• Assist with hygiene

Nutrition Optimization
• Set up tray and assist with feeding as needed
• Administer supplements
• Document nutritional intake

Discharge planning
• Assist with the assessment of psychosocial factors, including financial status and support systems
• Identify and report potential elder abuse
• Identify potential barriers to discharge
• Patient and family education on disease, medications, wound care, safety, and so forth.

delirium, including reorientation, providing hearing aids or glasses when possible, and environmental modifications for day/night differentiation.[33] Each of these interventions is performed most often by the nurse caring for the patient. Nurses can also help avoid the use of medications that contribute to delirium.

Nurses are uniquely able to identify psychosocial issues and barriers to discharge through daily interactions and developing relationships with the patient and family. Nurses observe the patient's mental status and gait throughout the duration of hospitalization and communicate these patterns to the medical provider and social worker. Family dynamics and support systems are often revealed through nurse interactions with the patient and family, and this information is helpful to facilitate a safe discharge plan. Nurses may also detect the potential for abuse, neglect, or self-neglect. Suspected abuse or neglect should be reported and may be mandatory depending on state laws.

CLINICS CARE POINTS

- Patients with geriatric trauma can have significant injuries even with low-energy mechanisms, such as falls.
- Blood thinners and antiplatelet medications increase the risk of life-threatening bleeding.
- Obtaining an accurate medical history and medication list is extremely important to identify risks and develop a comprehensive care plan.
- High-risk medications, such as anticholinergics and benzodiazepines, should be avoided in geriatric patients when possible.
- Patients with geriatric trauma with frailty have increased risk of poor outcomes, and multidisciplinary care can cost-effectively improve mortality, morbidity, functionality, LOS, and discharge disposition.
- The most effective delirium prevention measures are performed by the bedside nurse through environmental modifications, reorientation, and provision of hearing and vision aids.

DECLARATION OF INTERESTS

There are no commercial or financial conflicts of interests to disclose.

REFERENCES

1. Kozar RA, Arbabi S, Stein DM, et al. Injury in the aged: geriatric trauma care at the crossroads. J Trauma Acute Care Surg 2015;78(6):1197–209.
2. American College of Surgeons Committee on Trauma Leadership. National trauma Data Bank 2016 annual report. 2016 2016. Available at: https://www.facs.org/media/ez1hpdcu/ntdb-annual-report-2016.pdf. Accessed June 13,2022.
3. Bryant EA, Tulebaev S, Castillo-Angeles M, et al. Frailty identification and care pathway: an interdisciplinary approach to care for older trauma patients. J Am Coll Surg 2019;228:852–9.
4. Jacobs DG, Plaisier BR, Barie PS, et al. Practice management guidelines for geriatric trauma: the EAST practice management guidelines work group. J Trauma 2003;54:391–416.
5. Brooks SE, Peetz AB. Evidence-based care of geriatric trauma patients. Surg Clin North Am 2017;97:1157–74.

6. Clare D, Zink KL. Geriatric trauma. Emer Med Clin N Am 2021;39:257–71.
7. Maxwell CA, Patel MB, Suarez-Rodriguez LC, et al. Frailty and prognostication in geriatric surgery and trauma. Clin Geriatr Med 2019;35:13–26.
8. Yang R, Wolfson M, Lewis MC. Unique aspects of the elderly surgical population: an anesthesiologist's perspective. Geriatr Orthop Surg Rehabil 2011;2(2):56–64.
9. Brown JB, Gestring ML, Forsythe RM, et al. Systolic blood pressure criteria in the National Trauma Triage Protocol for geriatric trauma: 110 is the new 90. J Trauma Acute Care Surg 2015;78(2):352–9.
10. American Geriatrics Society 2019 Beers Criteria Update Expert Panel. American Geriatrics Society 2019 updated AGS Beers Criteria for potentially inappropriate medication use in older adults. J Am Geriatr Soc 2019;67:674–94.
11. Joseph B, Phelan H, Hassan A, et al. The impact of frailty on failure-to-rescue in geriatric trauma patients: a prospective study. J Trauma Acute Care Surg 2016; 81(6):1150–5.
12. Pecheva M, Phillips M, Hull P, et al. The impact of frailty in major trauma in older patients. Injury 2020;51:1536–42.
13. Poulton A, Shaw J, Nguyen F, et al. The association of frailty with adverse outcomes after multisystem trauma: a systematic review and meta-analysis. Anesth Analg 2020;130(6):1482–92.
14. Zhao F, Tang B, Hu C, et al. The impact of frailty on posttraumatic outcomes in older trauma patients: a systematic review and meta-analysis. J Trauma Acute Care Surg 2020;88(44):546–54.
15. McDonald VS, Thompson KA, Lewis PR, et al. Frailty in trauma: a systematic review of the surgical literature for clinical assessment tools. J Trauma Acute Care Surg 2016;80(5):824–34.
16. Cords CI, Spronk I, Mattace-Raso FUS, et al. The feasibility and reliability of frailty assessment tools applicable in acute in-hospital trauma patients: a systematic review. J Trauma Acute Care Surg 2022;92(3):615–26.
17. Jarman H, Crouch R, Baxter M, et al. Feasibility and accuracy of ED frailty identification in older trauma patients: a prospective multi-centre study. Scand J Trauma Resusc Emerg Med 2021;29:54.
18. Ma L, Tang Z, Chan P, et al. Novel frailty screening questionnaire (FSQ) predicts 8-year mortality in older adults. J Frailty Aging 2019;8(1):33–8.
19. Liu H, Shang N, Chhertri JK, et al. A frailty screening questionnaire (FSQ) to rapidly predict negative health outcomes of older adults in emergency care settings. J Nut Health Aging 2020;24(6):627–33.
20. Zhang Y, Zhang Y, Li Y, et al. Reliability and validity of the self-reported frailty screening questionnaire in older adults. Ther Adv Chronic Dis 2020;11:1–8.
21. Pincus D, Ravi R, Wasserstein D, et al. Association between wait time and 30-day mortality in adults undergoing hip fracture surgery. JAMA 2017;318(20): 1994–2003.
22. Folbert EC, Hegeman JH, Vermeer M, et al. Improved 1-year mortality in elderly patients with a hip fracture following integrated orthogeriatric treatment. Osteoporos Int 2017;28:269–77.
23. Wilson JM, Boissonneault AR, Schwartz AM, et al. Frailty and malnutrition are associated with inpatient postoperative complications and mortality in hip fracture patients. J Orthop Trauma 2019;33(3):143–8.
24. Moola S. Malnutrition risk (elderly): protein and energy supplementation. The Joanna Briggs Institute EBP Database; 2019. p. JBI1151.

25. Eamer G, Taheri A, Chen SS, et al. Comprehensive geriatric assessment for older people admitted to a surgical service. Cochrane Database Syst Rev 2018;1(1): CD012485.

26. American College of Surgeons. ACS TQIP geriatric trauma management guidelines. American College of Surgeons; 2013. Available at: https://www.facs.org/-/media/files/quality-programs/trauma/tqip/geriatric_guidelines.ashx.   Accessed August 22, 2022.

27. American College of Surgeons. Optimal resources for geriatric surgery: 2019 standards. American College of Surgeons; 2019. Available at: https://www.facs.org/-/media/files/quality-programs/geriatric/geriatricsv_standards.ashx.   Accessed August 22, 2022.

28. Katrancha ED, Zipf J, Abrahams N, et al. Retrospective evaluation of the impact of a geriatric trauma institute on fragility hip fracture patient outcomes. Orthop Nurs 2017;36(5):330–4.

29. Neuerburg C, Forch S, Gleich J, et al. Improved outcome in hip fracture patients in the aging population following co-managed care compared to conventional surgical treatment: a retrospective, dual-center cohort study. BMC Geriatr 2019;19(330). https://doi.org/10.1186/s12877-019-1289-6.

30. Prestmo A, Hagen G, Sletvold O, et al. Comprehensive geriatric care for patients with hip fractures: a prospective, randomized, controlled trial. Lancet 2015;325: 1623–33.

31. Engelhardt KE, Reuter O, Liu J, et al. Frailty screening and a frailty pathway decrease length of stay, loss of independence, and 30-day readmission rates in frail geriatric trauma and emergency general surgery patients. J Trauma Acute Care Surg 2018;85(1):167–73.

32. Slade S, Ther GDM. Frail elderly: multi-disciplinary management and social worker role. The Joanna Briggs Institute EBL Database; 2017. p. JB17312.

33. Siddiqi N, Harrison JK, Clegg A, et al. Interventions for preventing delirium in hospitalised non-ICU patients. Cochrane Database Syst Rev 2016;3:CD005563.

34. Gleich J, Pfeufer D, Zeckey C, et al. Orthogeriatric treatment reduces potential inappropriate medication in older trauma patients: a retrospective, dual-center study comparing conventional trauma care and co-managed treatment. Eur J Med Res 2019;24(4). https://doi.org/10.1186/s40001-019-0362-0.

35. Olufajo OA, Tulebaev S, Javedan H, et al. Integrating geriatric consults into routine care of older trauma patients: one-year experience of a level I trauma center. J Am Coll Surg 2016;222(6):1029–35.

Evidence-Based Pearls
Falls in the Intensive Care Unit

Alison H. Davis, PhD, RN, CNE, CHSE[a],*,
Aimme J. McCauley, DNP, MSN, RN, CNE[b]

KEYWORDS

- Critical care • Evidence-based bundle • Evidence-based prevention • Falls
- Intensive care • Risk assessment • Risk factors

KEY POINTS

- Intensive care unit (ICU)-acquired weakness, sedation, and environmental factors contribute to high risk for patient falls in the ICU.
- Hospital 30-day readmissions due to a fall after discharge are increasing globally, prompting focused attention on the impact of ICU-acquired weakness and family and caregiver engagement.
- Fall prevention and screening tools, bundles, and programs are most effective when tailored to patient specifics, such as age, length of stay, history of falls, mental status, and toileting needs.
- Family and caregiver education is of key importance in preventing inpatient falls, as well as readmission due to falls after discharge.

INTRODUCTION
Definitions

Patient falls are a major global health problem, affecting patients through their life span. Falls are prevalent in the intensive care units (ICUs) and are compounded by a myriad of factors from the pediatric to geriatric patient populations. The Joint Commission defines falls as "a fall may be described as an unintentional change in position coming to rest on the ground, floor, or onto the next lower surface."[1] However, the Joint Commission encourages health-care organizations to check their state guidelines as laws and/or regulations surrounding falls can provide differing definitions of a fall for states within the United States (US). The World Health Organization (WHO) takes a global lens and defines a fall as "an event which results in a person coming to rest inadvertently on the ground or floor or other lower level."[2]

[a] School of Nursing, Louisiana State University Health Sciences Center New Orleans, 1900 Gravier Street, #5A10, New Orleans, LA 70112, USA; [b] School of Nursing, Louisiana State University Health Sciences Center New Orleans, 1900 Gravier Street, #5B7, New Orleans, LA 70112, USA
* Corresponding author.
E-mail address: adav27@lsuhsc.edu

Crit Care Nurs Clin N Am 35 (2023) 161–170
https://doi.org/10.1016/j.cnc.2023.02.008
0899-5885/23/© 2023 Elsevier Inc. All rights reserved.

ccnursing.theclinics.com

Background/History

The incidence of patient falls in the acute care setting is estimated between 3.7 and 4.8 per 1000 patients per day in the adult patient population.[3] Pediatric patients fall at a rate of 0.56 to 2.19 per 1000 per day.[4] Falls contribute to patient injury and mortality. The WHO reports that falls are the second leading cause of injury and mortality globally, with an estimated 684,000 individuals dying from falls or fall-related injuries annually.[2] Falls are also the leading cause of nonfatal injuries in patients aged 65 years or older.

Falls can result in serious patient harm. As high as 50% of falls result in patient injury, with fractures, bruises, bleeding, and concussions reported as serious injuries because of a fall.[4] There is a paucity of research exploring the incidence of falls in the ICU to include vulnerable populations such as children and younger adults ($\leq$65 years of age). Hospitals may not collect data differentiating falls with injury from noninjurious falls. Lack of research surrounding patient falls, in general, may be due to an underreporting of fall occurrences due to feeling of guilt, negligence, fear, lack of a record system, concern over lawsuits, and intuitional cultures that promote avoidance of financial penalties.[5] Underreporting of falls proves research to be challenging in this area due to lack of data or insufficient data in certain patient populations.

Historically, patient falls have not been considered a major quality concern.[6] Healthcare providers are now recognizing that ICU treatment modalities are leading to patient immobility, resulting in ICU-acquired weakness. One immobility statistic reports that "patients spend more than 95% of their time in bed."[7] ICU-acquired weakness predicts post-ICU physical impairment to include overall functional status, return to work, overall quality of life, and institutionalization.[7,8] Falls in adults have been directly linked with ICU-acquired weakness or "posthospital syndrome"[7] and are considered an immediate patient risk factor associated with early mobility practices implemented in the ICU. The use of bed and chair alarms to prevent falls are cited as further restricting patient mobility and are ineffective to reduce patient falls. Bed and chair alarms are cited not only as ineffective but also as adding to health-care provider stress through alarm fatigue, especially for nurses, while increasing health-care costs due to associated falls and injury from falls.[7]

Falls result in increased hospital costs. Fall-related injury care has been estimated at more than US$30 billion annually in the adult population alone. Internationally, the human and financial costs of falls are gaining recognition because the impacts to patient outcomes are vast and even severe. Patients who fall are reported to stay an additional 8 days in the hospital setting.[9] The Centers for Medicare and Medicaid Services (CMS) identified conditions resulting in higher Medicare costs that were preventable with evidence-based care in 2007. As a result, in 2008 CMS executed new payment provisions. These provisions no longer reimbursed hospitals for hospital-acquired conditions, to include falls resulting in injury.[7] The Affordable Care Act also included financial penalties for hospitals with low hospital-acquired conditions beginning in 2010. Health-care costs associated with ICU admissions are substantial with mechanical ventilation as a significant contributor to overall costs. Daily rates for an ICU admission have been reported from approximately US$1000 to US$1500 depending on patient acuity.[10] The additional of an unintentional fall has been reported to cost an average of US$7000 per patient per day in the ICU.[9]

DISCUSSION
Fall Risk in the Intensive Care Unit

Patients admitted to the ICU are noted to be at a high risk for falls. Patients are falling in the ICU due to immobility related to diagnoses necessitating complex treatment modalities. In 2022, the incidence rates of falls in the ICU was reported as "9.7/1000 (95% CI, 8.95–10.37) per patient admitted to an ICU and 1.78 falls per 1000 (95% CI, 1.65–1.91) patient days in the ICU."[6] Immobility is directly related to weakness. The frequency of falls is reported to increase with each day spent in the ICU. Falls in the ICU are being examined to understand risks for falls, other than medical diagnosis and sedating medications.

Patients admitted to ICUs are being studied to assist health-care providers to understand the incidence and causes of falls. Most patients in the ICU are mechanically ventilated and receive vasopressors. Intensive care admissions vary and include, but are not limited to, postoperative major surgery, acute respiratory distress, septic shock, and posttrauma. This variety of admissions has led to younger patients (aged younger than 65 years) with more complex diagnoses. Patient who are aged younger than 65 years, admitted from the emergency department, have a medical admission, have higher Acute Physiology and Chronic Health Evaluation (APACHE) and Sequential Organ Failure Assessment (SOFA) scores, receive mechanical ventilation, require dialysis, experience delirium, and the number of mobilizations have been reported as related to an increased risk for falling in the ICU.[6,11] In addition, impaired walking ability, being unaccompanied, anticoagulant and/or sedative use, decreased strength, slipping, tripping, fainting, and seizures are characteristics of patients who are at increased risk of falls while in the ICU.[3] Environmental factors can contribute to patient falls to include equipment failure, wet areas (floors), lack of bed rails in the up position, poor lighting, obstacles, and newly waxed floors.[3] If a patient fell, they were almost 8% likely to fall again, and almost 2% likely to fall 3 or more times while in the ICU.[6]

Characteristics of falls vary in the ICU regarding location and time. The majority of falls are noted to happen in the daytime, with 25% occurring between 10 PM and 6 AM Most patients fell from bed (29.7%), chair (19.9%), or during patient mobilization (23.9%) and were witnessed by a member of the health-care team.[6] Restrained patients are not immune from falls. One study noted that 10.6% of patients were reported as falling while restrained.[6]

Early mobility (EM) practices are designed to "optimize ICU patient outcomes."[8] There are risks associated with EM, including falls. Patient falls during EM are associated with ICU-acquired weakness secondary to immobility. Nurses are noted as the main initiators of EM in ICU patients, second to physical therapists. Additionally, if a nurse makes a decision that EM is inappropriate for an ICU patient, EM will likely not take place.

Early mobilization can be affected by situational or environmental factors. Low staffing is a major reason for delaying or not performing EM as reported by nurses and physical therapists. These providers reported feeling unsafe to ambulate an ICU patient alone as EM should be a team activity.[8] Workload contributes to EM. Because EM should be a team effort, inconvenience can hinder the process because not all team members are available at the same time. Additionally, the more equipment and monitors that a patient has for their care, the less likely EM will occur due to management of these items. A lack of mobility or patient lifting equipment can also prevent EM because health-care providers need resources to safely facilitate EM.

Health-care providers, especially nurses and physical therapists, have reported understanding the long-term benefits of EM for ICU patients but are cautious due to the immediate patient risks.[8] Immediate risks have been reported as "acute decomposition" and "always risk of patient fall."[8] Early mobilization practices have shown improved mobility outcomes for ICU patients. However, EM and the association with a patient's risk of falls have not been studied widely in the ICU setting.

Evidence-Based Prevention Strategies for Fall Prevention

Early identification of patients who are at an increased risk of falls in the ICU is critical for preventing falls. Implementation of clinical best practices and comprehensive fall prevention and safety programs are essential for ICUs. Clinical best practice guidelines are comprehensive documents that serve as to enhance decision-making, in this case, surrounding falls in adult patients. These guidelines prove resources for evidence-based practice for nurses and health-care providers. A fall prevention and safety program should be initiated on admission to an ICU. Evidence-based assessment tools, scales, and guides are methods to screen and identify high-risk patients in the ICU setting. Following the screening, protective measures can be used for increased patient safety and positive outcomes, including decreased mortality resulting from a fall. However, there is disagreement surrounding screening tools. The effectiveness of "any screening tool"[12] is unclear to predict or prevent falls in the hospital. Fall screening tools are noted to have varied performance depending on the hospital setting.

Historically, fall prevention screening tools and guides focus on the elderly because of this population's increased risk of falls. Recently, context specific tools have been cited as more effective than the risk-assessment tools at preventing falls. A discussion of evidence-based fall risk-assessment tools and guides will ensue. This discussion will provide evidence to assist health-care providers to reduce falls in the ICU patient. Major components for the fall prevention and risk-assessment tools are located in **Table 1**.

Fall Prevention and Risk-Assessment Tools

Morse Fall Scale. The Morse Fall Scale was developed to estimate the risk of patient falls in a variety of settings. The authors recommend the scale be calibrated to the local population being assessed to ensure prevention strategies are tailored to the specific patients. Tailoring the scale captures the fact that the risk of falls varies according to the type of patient, different times of day, and in different situations a patient may be exposed to while under a provider's care.[13] Unfortunately, critical patients score high on the scale due to their characteristics, such as impaired gait due to weakness or presence of an intravenous lock.[3]

ONTARIO Modified STRATIFY. The ONTARIO Modified STRATIFY (OM) Falls Risk Screen (ONTARIO) is used to screen elderly patients for falls. The ONTARIO is adapted from the STRATIFY tool to increase the sensitivity and specificity to older patients. The OM includes 6 domains for fall risk assessment. A risk score of 9 or greater indicates patients at a higher risk of falling. This tool includes a list of care actions that are applicable to all patients and a link to provide families with fall risk prevention information.

Northern Hospital Modified STRATIFY Tool. The Northern Hospital Modified STRATIFY (TNH) tool was developed to increase the sensitivity and specificity of the STRATIFY for use in older patients. This tool is similar to STRATIFY but separates hospital falls and falls within the last year. Nine items are included and a score of 3 or more indicates high risk of falling. Operational definitions are included for each item. The tool requires daily patient assessment and findings can be integrated into the plan of care.

STRATIFY Tool. This tool was developed to identify fall risk factors in hospitalized patients. STRATIFY includes 5 items for predicting hospital falls. Two or more positive answers indicate a patient is high risk for falls. This tool has been reported as having high specificity for elderly patients at risk of falling.[12] Items in the tool have been noted to be easily and quickly assessed by nurses and requires little to no training. A limitation of the tool is reported as the outcomes of the tool is falls and not patients who at risk for falling.

Table 1 Fall prevention and risk assessment tools components		
Tool or Scale	**Characteristics**	**Limitations**
Morse Fall Scale	• Developed for hospitalized clinical patient • Six domains: history of falling, secondary diagnosis, ambulatory aid, IV/Heparin lock, gait/transferring, mental status • Scores range: 0–125 • Higher scores = higher risk of falling	• Critical patients score high routinely on the scale
ONTARIO Modified STRATIFY (OM)	• Six domains: history of falls, mental status, vision, toileting, transfer, mobility	• Often used in conjunction with a risk level intervention guide
STRATIFY	• Five items: presentation to hospital with fall or a fall since admission, agitation, visual impairment affecting activities of daily living, need for frequent toileting, transfer and mobility score of 3 or 4 on the Barthel index	• Specificity for elderly patients
Northern Hospital Modified STRATIFY Tool	• Nine items: falls (current admission); fall in last 12 mo; confused, disoriented, intellectually challenged, agitated or has impulsive behavior; needs supervision or assistance with mobility; impaired balance or hemiplegia; ≥80 y; frequent toileting; visually impaired with affect to everyday functioning; presented with drug-related or alcohol-related issues	• Requires daily patient assessment

Strategy bundles and programs are available to prevent falls in and after discharge from the hospital setting. A discussion of the ABCDEF strategy, Hospital Elder Life Program (HELP), and Stopping Elderly Accidents, Deaths, and Injuries (STEADI) Program is included in the following paragraphs.

ABCDEF Strategy. The ABCDEF strategy is an evidence-based bundle designed to guide strategies to reduce falls. The strategy includes "*A*ssess, Prevent, and Manage Pain, *B*oth Spontaneous Awakening Trials and Spontaneous Breathing Trials (SBT), *C*hoice of analgesia and sedation, *D*elirium: Assess, Prevent, and Manage, *E*arly mobility and Exercise, and *F*amily engagement and empowerment."[14] Early mobility is a component of the ABCDEF interprofessional team strategy to manage critically ill patients. Collaboration is facilitated among health-care professionals while standardizing ICU processes.[8] Early mobility has been cited as the most difficult component of the bundle to implement due to various reasons. Reasons have been identified such as immediate patient risks (falls), hemodynamic instability, and dislodgment of equipment/lines (extracorporeal membrane oxygenation [ECMO] cannula, chest tubes, central lines).[8]

Hospital Elder Life Program. This program is considered an innovative model of hospital care for older adults.[15] The interprofessional team is the focus of this tool to enhance patient mobility while decreasing falls. However, volunteers are instrumental for the program and focus on providing supportive care and attention to elderly patients. The program is designed to prevent delirium, a leading risk factor for falls. The HELP contains multiple components for fall reduction and has shown efficacy in practice.[7] The program goals include "Maintaining cognitive and physical functioning of high risk older adults throughout hospitalization; Maximizing independence at discharge; Assisting with the transition from hospital to home; and Preventing unplanned hospital readmissions."[15]

STEADI Program. The Centers for Disease Control (CDC) developed STEADI as a fall prevention program. The STEADI program was an initiative than then transitioned by the CDC to become the CDC STEADI: Best Practices for Developing an Inpatient Program to Prevent Older Adult Falls after Discharge. This guide was developed for health-care providers to evaluate and assess patients for falls before and after discharge. The guide is free and is a systematic, evidence-based resource for managing falls and assessing fall risks. STEADI uses an algorithm to assess fall risk, tips for integrating fall risk management into clinical practice, assessment tools for modifiable fall-risk factors, descriptions of interventions, and patient education materials. The guide includes 10 steps designed to "decrease patient falls during and after hospital stays; promote better collaboration with external providers for postdischarge care; improve hospital processes and records; and identify and manage medications that increase patient falls."[16]

Clinical Best Practice Guideline

Clinical practice guidelines are developed for use by health-care professionals. These guidelines summarize current medical knowledge, analyze risks and benefits of diagnostic procedures and treatments, and provide evidence-based recommendations that are specific to a topic.[17] Information about scientific evidence is included to support recommendations and is graded according to the strength of the level of evidence of the research. A description of a clinical practice guideline aimed at preventing falls and reducing injury from falls will follow.

Preventing Falls and Reducing Injury From Falls. Developed by the Registered Nurses' Association of Ontario (RNAO), this guideline was designed to provide excellence in clinical care, leading to excellent patient health outcomes, communities, and the health-care system.[18] Nurses who provide direct clinical care to adults at risk of falling are the intended audience for the guideline's practice recommendations. This

---

Box 1
Guiding principles for preventing falls and reducing injury from falls[18]

- Many falls are predictable and preventable.
- Some falls cannot be prevented; in these cases, the focus should be on proactively preventing fall injuries and decreasing the frequency of falls.
- Falls prevention is a shared responsibility within health care.
- Person-centered and family-centered care is foundational to the care of people at risk for falls and fall injuries.
- The risks and benefits for the person should be considered when implementing interventions to prevent falls and minimize injuries.
- Competent adults have the right to take risks (ie, make decisions or take actions that increase their risk for falls).

denotes the importance of nurses in the prevention of falls. A secondary audience includes members of the interprofessional team. The guideline is for use in adults aged 18 years or older who are at a risk of falling in the health-care environment (primary care, home health care, acute care, and long-term care settings). The guideline is not recommended for preventing falls in the population-level, workplace, industry, and children or for intentional falls, sports-related falls, and building designs. Six principles are cited as guidelines for the document. These principles are included in **Box 1**.

The practice recommendations for the guideline are summarized in **Box 2**. provides the flow chart for falls prevention and injury reduction.

Box 2
Practice recommendations: preventing falls and reducing injury from falls summary[18]

Practice Recommendations
Recommendation 1.0:
- Screen all adults to identify those at risk for falls.
- For adults at risk for falls, conduct a comprehensive assessment to identify factors contributing to risk and determine appropriate interventions.
- Refer adults with recurrent falls, multiple risk factors, or complex needs to the appropriate clinician(s) or to the interprofessional team.
Recommendation 2.0:
- Engage adults at risk for falls and fall injuries.
- Provide education to the person at risk for falls and fall injuries and their family.
- Communicate the person's risk for falls and related plan of care/interventions to the next responsible health-care provider and/or the interprofessional team at all care transitions.
- Implement a combination of interventions.
- Recommend exercise interventions and physical training for adults at risk for falls.
- Collaborate with prescribers and the person at risk for falls to reduce, gradually withdraw, or discontinue medications that are associated with falling.
- Refer adults at risk for falls or fall injuries to the appropriate health-care provider for advice about vitamin D supplementation.
- Encourage dietary interventions and other strategies to optimize bone health.
- Consider hip protectors as an intervention to reduce the risk of hip fracture.
Recommendation 3.0:
After a person falls, provide the following interventions:
- Physical examination to assess for injury and to determine the severity.
- Provide appropriate treatment and care.
- Monitor for injuries.
- Conduct a postfall assessment.
- Collaborate with the person and the interprofessional team to conduct further assessments.
- Refer the person to the appropriate health-care provider(s) for physical rehabilitation and/or to support psychological well-being.

Education Recommendations
Recommendation 4.0:
- Educational institutions incorporate content on falls prevention and injury reduction.
- Health-care organizations provide ongoing organization-wide education to all staff.

Organization and Policy Recommendations
Recommendation 5.0:
- Ensure a safe environment
  ○ Implement universal falls precautions, and to identify and modify equipment and other factors in the physical/structural environment.
- Organizational leaders, in collaboration with teams, apply implementation science strategies to enable successful implementation and sustainability of falls prevention/injury reduction initiatives.
- Implement rounding.

The RNAO recommends implementing the Preventing Falls and Reducing Injury From Falls guideline by adapting the guideline to individual practice settings, ensuring a good fit for the local context. The guidelines are best adopted using the RNAO Toolkit: Implementation of Best Practice Guidelines, which uses the Knowledge-to-Action (KTA) framework. Implementing the guideline based on the process steps of the KTA framework ensures adaption on new knowledge while identifying any gaps in a particular setting.

Evaluation strategies and measures are provided in the Preventing Falls and Reducing Injury from Falls guideline. These data repositories as well as instruments include the following:

Nursing Quality Indicators for Reporting and Evaluation, Canadian Institutes for Health Information Continuing Care Reporting System, The Resident Assessment Instrument Minimum Data Set Version 2.0, The interRAI–Acute Care, Canadian Institute for Health Information Home Care Reporting System, Ontario Association of Community Care Access Centers Home Care Database, The Resident Assessment Instrument–Home Care, The interRAI–Contact Assessment, Canadian Institute for Health Information Discharge Abstract Database, Canadian- Health Outcomes for Better Information and Care, Canadian Institute for Health Information National Ambulatory Care Reporting System, Canadian Institute for Health Information Ontario Trauma Registry, and Canadian Institute for Health Information Hospital Mortality Database.[18]

Through evaluation of fall prevention strategies, determination of whether the strategies are a good fit for the local context can be completed. This will assist with applicability for patient care and promote positive patient outcomes as falls and fall risks are reduced.

SUMMARY

Falls are multifaceted and can affect patients of all ages in all hospital settings, including ICUs. Patients aged older than 65 years are noted to have between a 5.5% and 24.8% chance of falling while hospitalized.[12] However, younger patients (<65 years of age) are falling in the ICU. Falls experienced by patients aged younger than 65 years are being contributed to immobility and resulting weakness. Additionally, immobility has been noted as contributing to falls in patients aged 65 years or older, but older age has historically been determined as a high risk of falling while hospitalized. Risk factors for falls in the ICU include higher APACHE and SOFA scores, mechanical ventilation, dialysis, delirium, impaired walking ability, being unaccompanied, anticoagulant and/or sedative use, decreased strength, slipping, tripping, fainting, and seizures along with total number of mobilizations.[6,11]

Evidence-based fall prevention and screening tools along with implementation of clinical practice guidelines specific to falls can decrease the overall rate of falls in the ICU. These tools need to be assessed for local context, although, ensuring they are applicable to the current, specific patient population. Using these tools and guidelines, patient outcomes surrounding falls can be improved, resulting in less unintentional injury for patients who are hospitalized.

CLINICS CARE POINTS

- Competent adults have the right to take risks but many falls can be prevented.
- The most-effective fall prevention strategies are tailored to the patient, are patient and family-centered, and recognize that fall prevention is a shared responsibility within health care.

- ICU patients should be assessed for fall risk daily because fall risk increases with length of stay in critical care settings.
- Evidence-based bundles for falls prevention, such as the ABCDEF Strategy, should be implemented for patients at high risk for falls while in the hospital setting.
- For patients at high risk for falls after discharge, evidence-based bundles for falls prevention, such as the STEADI Program, should be implemented.

DECLARATION OF INTERESTS

The authors have nothing to disclose.

REFERENCES

1. Fall reduction program - definition and resources | critical access hospital | provision of care treatment and Services PC | the Joint commission. Available at: https://www.jointcommission.org/standards/standard-faqs/critical-access-hospital/provision-of-care-treatment-and-services-pc/000002150. Accessed October 19, 2022.
2. World Health Organization. Falls. Falls. Available at: https://www.who.int/newsroom/fact-sheets/detail/falls. Accessed October 20, 2022.
3. Martins Specht A, Peres De Sousa G, Gomes Beghetto M. Online Revista Gaúcha de Enfermagem Incidence of falls in a cohort of critical adults: a cause for concerns? Rev Gaúcha Enferm 2020;41:20190167.
4. AlSowailmi BA, AlAkeely MH, AlJutaily HI, et al. Prevalence of fall injuries and risk factors for fall among hospitalized children in a specialized children's hospital in Saudi Arabia. Ann Saudi Med 2018;38(3):225.
5. Evangelou E, Associate R, Middleton N, et al. Nursing quality indicators for adult intensive care: a consensus study. Nurs Crit Care 2020. https://doi.org/10.1111/nicc.12543.
6. Wu G, Soo A, Ronksley P, et al. A multicenter cohort study of falls among patients admitted to the ICU. Crit Care Med 2022;50(5):810–8.
7. Growdon ME, Shorr RI, Inouye SK. The tension between promoting mobility and preventing falls in the Hospital. JAMA Intern Med 2017;177(6):759–60.
8. Boehm LM, Lauderdale J, Garrett AN, et al. A multisite study of multidisciplinary ICU team member beliefs toward early mobility. Heart Lung 2021. https://doi.org/10.1016/j.hrtlng.2020.09.021.
9. Tyndall A, Bailey R, Elliott R. Pragmatic development of an evidence-based intensive care unitespecific falls risk assessment tool: the Tyndall Bailey Falls Risk Assessment Tool. Aust Crit Care 2019. https://doi.org/10.1016/j.aucc.2019.02.003.
10. Kaier K, Heister T, Wolff J, et al. Mechanical ventilation and the daily cost of ICU care. BMC Health Serv Res 2020;20(1):1–5.
11. Patman SM, Cert G, Teaching U, et al. The incidence of falls in intensive care survivors. Aust Crit Care 2011;24:167–74.
12. Latt MD, Loh KF, Ge L, et al. The validity of three fall risk screening tools in an acute geriatric inpatient population. Australas J Ageing 2016;35(3):167–73.
13. Morse JM, Tylko SJ, Dixon HA. Characteristics of the fall-prone patient. Gerontologist 1987;27(4):516–22.

14. Marra A, Ely EW, Pandharipande PP, et al. The ABCDEF bundle in critical care HHS public access. Crit Care Clin 2017;33(2):225–43.
15. Hospital elder life program | hinda and arthur marcus Institute for aging research. Available at: https://www.marcusinstituteforaging.org/research/aging-brain-center/hospital-elder-life-program-help. Accessed October 19, 2022.
16. Inpatient care | STEADI - older adult fall prevention | CDC injury center. Available at: https://www.cdc.gov/steadi/inpatient-care.html. Accessed October 17, 2022.
17. What are clinical practice guidelines? - InformedHealth.org - NCBI Bookshelf. Available at: https://www.ncbi.nlm.nih.gov/books/NBK390308/?report=reader. Accessed October 19, 2022.
18. Registered Nurses' Association of Ontario. (2017). Preventing falls and reducing injury from falls (4th ed.). Toronto, ON. https://rnao.ca/sites/rnao-ca/files/bpg/FALL_PREVENTION_WEB_1207-17.pdf. Accessed October 18, 2022.

Evidence-Based Pearls
Traumatic Brain Injury

Mary Ritter, DNP, MSN, MLS, APRN, FNPBC[a,b,*]

KEYWORDS

- Head injury • Traumatic brain injury • Evidence-based pearls • Nursing management
- Intracranial hypertension • Treatment strategies • Rehabilitation • Brain trauma

KEY POINTS

- Evidence-based pearls in the management of traumatic brain injury.
- Management with operative and non-operative interventions.
- More focus on non-operative management to reduce mortality.

Traumatic brain injury (TBI) is an injury to the brain resulting from a sudden jolt, bump, or another direct impact on the head leading to alterations in brain function. In the United States, over 2.2 million individuals present to emergency departments seeking treatment of TBI. Of the 2.2 million, approximately 283,000 were treated and discharged from the emergency department.[1] However, over 52,000 of the 2.2 million will succumb to TBI. The highest rates of TBI occur in young children (0–4 years old), adolescents (15–24 years old), and the elderly (over 65 years old).[2] TBI is more common in men than women. It is the leading cause of death and disability in children and adolescents. The most common causes of TBI in the United States include falls and motor vehicle accidents.[3]

The severity of TBI is classified as mild, moderate, or severe. Classification is determined by presenting clinical manifestations. Moderate to severe TBI may result in permanent disability or functional alterations with persistent symptoms, even death. Mild TBI may result in transient effects. The severity of the injury is directly related to the type of external impact resulting in TBI. The severity of TBI further determines the level of impact on the quality of life faced by the affected individual. TBI is a leading cause of death in the United States. Individuals with TBI (even mild TBI) have a significantly increased risk of death when compared with those in the general population.[3]

A large number of TBIs occurring annually are mild TBIs, resulting from trauma that causes the brain/head to move quickly backward and forward.[4] The backward and

---

[a] Southeastern Louisiana University, Hammond, LA, USA; [b] Urgent Care, Premier Health, Baton Rouge, LA, USA
* 4950 Essen Lane, Baton Rouge, LA 70809.
E-mail address: mritterdnp@gmail.com

Crit Care Nurs Clin N Am 35 (2023) 171–178
https://doi.org/10.1016/j.cnc.2023.02.009
0899-5885/23/© 2023 Elsevier Inc. All rights reserved.

ccnursing.theclinics.com

forward rapid motion of the head causes chemical alterations in the brain tissue and stretching of brain cells with ultimate damage to the involved brain cells. TBI is classified as mild, moderate, or severe (**Table 1**), further classified as (1) closed brain injury and (2) penetrating brain injury.[5] Any TBI is considered a "serious" injury, even mild TBIs. Neurologic exams will usually facilitate the identification of any worrisome signs or symptoms. Mild TBI does not warrant a computerized tomography (CT) scan. Common signs and/or symptoms include headache, confusion, dizziness, ringing in the ears, blurry vision, changes in behavior, and intermittent memory loss or impairment.[5]

Moderate TBI may be the direct result of a penetrating injury (such as a gunshot wound), sudden jolt, bump, or blow to the head. Common signs and/or symptoms include vomiting, slurred speech, extremity weakness, issues with learning or memory, confusion, seizures, and possible death.[4]

Severe TBI is caused by a penetrating injury direct blow, sudden jolt, or bump to the head, which also results in prolonged loss of consciousness. Long-term consequences are varied from intermittent to permanent deficits in cognitive, motor, and/or sensory function, and possible psychiatric alterations. Common signs and/or symptoms include persistent or worsening headache, vomiting, slurred speech, extremity weakness, issues with learning or memory, convulsions/seizures, dilation of one or both pupils, difficulty arousing, and possible death.[4]

CLINICAL RELEVANCE AND DIAGNOSTICS

Long-term complications associated with TBI include epilepsy, neurodegenerative disorders, sleep disorders, Alzheimer's disease, chronic traumatic encephalopathy, post-traumatic hypopituitarism, psychiatric disorders, incontinence, sexual dysfunction, musculoskeletal dysfunction, and metabolic dysfunction.[2] The associated long-term complications are directly correlated with the severity of reduced cerebral blood flow resulting from TBI. Damage may be focal or diffuse depending on the type of injury to the brain. The impact of such complications on quality of life and

Table 1
Traumatic brain injury

Degree	Characteristics
Mild	Minimal (less than a few minutes or seconds) loss of consciousness, or no loss of consciousness; May appear confused or disoriented; other symptoms: headaches, intermittent memory loss, attention or concentration difficulty Results from sudden movements (such as shaking head or rapid change in motion-"Whiplash")
Moderate	Loss of consciousness for a period of hours with confusion or disorientation lasting week; Physical, sensory, cognitive, and behavioral complications may be present (may last for weeks);
Severe	Life threatening (Usually results from a crush or penetration injury to the head); Maybe a closed or open injury to the skull; common injuries resulting in severe TBI include skull fracture resulting from slip and fall, gunshot wound to the head, motor vehicle accidents, sports-related injuries as a direct result from excessive force; significant cognitive, physical, sensory, and/or behavioral complications may be present (may be transient or permanent)

From Centers for Disease Control. (2022). Traumatic brain injury and concussion. Retrieved from: https://www.cdc.gov/traumaticbraininjury/index.html.

functional ability may be life-altering or life-limiting. Costs associated with TBI exceed $40 billion annually in health care, significantly greater when lost wages are considered.

Diagnosing TBI may be complicated if symptoms are vague, as in a mild TBI. Physical exam facilitates the identification of signs and symptoms associated with TBI.[5] A thorough physical exam with an extensive neurologic evaluation is required to sufficiently assess and identify a TBI and degree of injury. Imaging may help to identify brain injury (**Box 1**). CT scans and MRI are often beneficial in accurately identifying TBI and establishing the degree of injury. Imaging also facilitates determining the need for surgical intervention. Other diagnostic testing which may help to accurately identify TBI include serum laboratory testing (complete blood count, coagulation profile, metabolic panel, and arterial blood gases); radiograph images (skull and cervical spine); intracranial pressure monitor; Glasgow Coma Scale; and vital signs. Clinical manifestations exhibited by the patient will assist with the diagnosis of TBI and facilitate the evaluation of response to treatment.

NON-OPERATIVE TREATMENT

Conservative management of TBI focuses on achieving and maintaining hemodynamic stability via the use of non-operative interventions. Many of these interventions are effective and less costly when compared with operative interventions in the management of TBI. Patient positioning with head in a neutral position and head of bed elevated at 30° to facilitate cerebral venous drainage and prevent increased intracranial pressure.[6] Supplemental oxygenation to maintain oxygen saturation levels at 93% or greater, promotes oxygenation of brain tissue and decreases mortality.[7]

Sedatives and/or analgesics are used to maintain a calm, steady state, preventing increased intracranial pressure. Anticonvulsants, such as phenytoin, may be administered to prevent or control seizure activity.[7] Antihypertensive medications are administered to control blood pressure and prevent increased intracranial pressure. Other

---

Box 1
Diagnostics in traumatic brain injury

Physical Exam Findings
- Vital signs for hemodynamic stability
- Systematic neurologic exam
  - Glasgow Coma Scale
- Intracranial pressure monitor

Laboratory Testing
- Complete blood count, coagulation profile, metabolic panel, arterial blood gases

Radiograph Images
- Cervical Spine and Skull (to evaluate/identify fractures or displacement)

CT Scan
- High accuracy to identify injury and determining the extent of injury (grading)

MRI
- Rapid evaluation, non-invasive, inexpensive
- High specificity, low sensitivity
- Do not use exclusively for diagnosis

Adapted from Modello, S., Muller, U., Jeromin, A., Streeter, J., Hayes, R., & Wang, K. (2011). Blood-based diagnositics of traumatic brain injury. Expert molecular diagnostics, 11 (1), 65-78. Retrieved from: https://doi.org/10.1586/erm.10.104.

medications, such as calcium channel antagonists, magnesium, amino-steroids, and mannitol are administered to control swelling of the brain tissue, which assist with preventing increased intracranial pressure.[8] Steroids are not recommended as a therapeutic regimen in patients with TBI. Erythropoietin use has also demonstrated positive impact in improving neurologic outcomes and reducing mortality in TBI. Body temperature maintained in a hypothermic state facilitates a reduction in intracranial pressure.[4]

Individuals who have TBI will be in a hypermetabolic state immediately following the injury. To promote return to a normal metabolic state and support healing, enteral nutrition must be initiated within 72 hours of TBI.[5] Nutritional supplementation should include 1 to 1.5 g/kg for 2 weeks immediately following TBI. Intravenous fluid infusion will facilitate volume replacement, tissue perfusion, and restoration of vascular capacity. Isotonic intravenous solutions, such as normal saline, may be used if the patient is in a euvolemic state. If the patient with a TBI has septic shock or severe TBI, hypertonic solutions may be infused to support the patient.[6]

OPERATIVE MANAGEMENT

Surgical evacuation is considered a first-line treatment in patients with TBI and intracranial hematomas and Glasgow Coma Scale 8 or less.[7] If the intracranial hematoma is 30 mL or greater or the patient has a midline shift greater than 5 mm, surgical evacuation should occur regardless of the Glasgow Coma Scale.[9] Post-operative management requires close observation with continuous monitoring of intracranial pressure, cerebral perfusion, and cerebral spinal fluid circulation. Mechanical ventilation will assist with oxygenation, cerebral perfusion, and body temperature at a normal state.[7]

COMPLICATIONS

Patients with TBI are at risk for numerous complications depending on the degree of severity of TB.[10] Complications may involve one or numerous body systems, such as cardiovascular, respiratory, neurologic, and hematologic. Over 80% of patients with severe TBI will experience multi-system complications.[6] Possible complications of TBI are reviewed in **Table 2**.

NURSING CONSIDERATIONS

Priority goals for nursing care of patients with TBI include airway maintenance and achieving and maintaining cerebral perfusion. Maintaining hemodynamic stability is the central focus of nursing management in TBI patients.[9] Vital signs and physical assessments with thorough neurologic exams for complications should be completed frequently.[11] Pupillary response, corneal reflex, eye opening, gag reflex, sensation, motor strength, cognitive functioning, behavioral changes, and presence of vomiting or headache should be included in the neurologic examination. The symmetry of responses should also be assessed when conducting the physical examination.[6]

Close observation for the presence of deep vein thrombosis, secondary brain injury, or other complications related to TBI allows for early recognition and intervention. Supportive care and frequent nursing interventions will facilitate achieving and maintaining homeostasis. Common nursing interventions for TBI include head-of-bed elevation, seizure prophylaxis, hyperventilation, hyperosmolar medications, therapeutic cooling, medically-induced coma, intracranial pressure monitoring, and assessing for complications related to TBI.[11]

Table 2
Complications in traumatic brain injury[1]

Complications	Definition/Patho	Symptoms/Presentation	Treatment
Seizures	Sudden-onset disorganized brain activity resulting in jerking movements, dizziness, lip smacking More common with moderate or severe TBI May occur within 24 h of TBI or y following TBI More common when frontal or temporal lobe is involved in TBI.	Jerking movements, dizziness, loss of consciousness, lip smacking, repetitive movements.	Seizure precautions; Administration of phenytoin or levetiracetam.
Sepsis	Systemic inflammation resulting from chemicals released from brain to eliminate infection; widespread inflammation leads to multi-organ failure	Fever, hypotension (low blood pressure), rapid heart rate, difficulty breathing (possible ARDs or respiratory failure), confusion, weakness.	Analgesics; anti-pyretic medication (acetaminophen), intravenous fluid administration, antibiotic administration, supportive care. Overall goal to decrease sympathetic response.
Persistent sympathetic storming	Sympathetic hyperactivity Associated with a higher rate of mortality	Increased heart rate, blood pressure and respiratory rate; sweating; hyperthermia; motor posturing;	Administration of sedatives, opiate receptor antagonists, beta-blockers and/or Central Nervous System (CNS) depressants.
Increased intracranial pressure	Cerebral spinal fluid in ventricles increased, edema to brain tissue	Headache, cognitive decline, motor posturing, death;	Mannitol, hypertonic intravenous solution administration; head of bed at 30°, supportive care.
Vascular or cranial nerve injuries	May involve a single cranial nerve or multiple cranial nerves	Visual deficits, persistent ringing in ears (tinnitus), paresthesia of skin, abnormal or difficulty smelling	Rehabilitation therapy;
Sleep/wake disorders	Structural and biochemical alterations of brain Daytime napping	Inability to fall asleep and/or stay asleep	Sleep hygiene. Administration of benzodiazepines (such as lorazepam);sedatives (such as zolpidem); or melatonin Light therapy Exercise

(continued on next page)

Table 2
(continued)

Complications	Definition/Patho	Symptoms/Presentation	Treatment
Diffuse axonal injury	More severe form of TBI; resulting from shearing of brain tissue following shifting or rotation of brain inside the skull Usual results from blunt trauma to head Widespread injury to brain	Symptoms based on area of brain damage; Memory loss, confusion, lethargy, difficulty problem solving, decreased awareness of self and/or others, unable to understand abstract concepts, difficulty with time or special recognition, spasticity, weakness, paralysis, poor coordination, difficulty swallowing, one-sided neglect, visual deficits, aphasia, agraphia, inability to perform adls, comatose state	May require rehabilitation for y; safety precautions; administration of corticosteroids, anti-inflammatory medications
Chronic traumatic encephalopathy	Results from mild, recurrent TBI; unable to formally diagnose until brain biopsy on autopsy	Mood changes, worsening confusion; short-term memory loss; disorientation; difficulty with thinking and decision making, dysphagia, slurred speech	Supportive care; occupational, speech therapy
Respiratory failure	Proinflammatory state of TBI precipitates direct, significant endothelial destruction Multifactorial, dependent on degree of TBI	Hypoxia, pulmonary edema, acute respiratory distress syndrome (ARDs),	Aggressive treatment of TBI, mechanical ventilation, oxygen titration, optimal Positive End-Expiratory Pressure (PEEP), administration of neuromuscular blocking agents

Adapted from Ahmed, S., Venigalla, H., Mekala, H., Dar, S., Hassan, & Ayub, S. (2017). Traumatic brain injury and neuropsychiatric complications. Indian psychiatric society. Retrieved from: https://journals.sagepub.com/doi/pdf/10.4103/0253-7176.203129.

CASE STUDY

A 20-year-old woman presented to the emergency department after being ejected from the back of her boyfriend's motorcycle at high speed. The patient was wearing a helmet at impact. On exam, she was unresponsive in a prone with dilated pupils bilat, GCS 7, and numerous abrasions to the body surface area. The CT scan demonstrated a large subarachnoid hemorrhage with right frontal lobe involvement with a 2 mm midline shift and effacement of the ventricles. She was bradycardic with a pulse of 48 bpm, blood pressure 192/102 mm Hg, and respiratory rate of 28 breaths/min. A hypertonic solution of sodium chloride was initiated in the emergency department as a continuous infusion. Mannitol 30 mg was administered intravenously. Intracranial pressure was 4 and cerebral perfusion pressure was 75 mm Hg. She was transferred to the intensive care unit. On day 2 of hospitalization, the patient's head of the bed was moved to 45°. She had a sudden increase in intracranial pressure with motor posturing. The nurse entered the room to discover the patient experiencing motor posturing and realized the head of the bed was at 45°. The nurse corrected the bed position, placing the head of the bed at 30° and evaluated the patient's vital signs and neurologic status. The nurse notified the physician of the patient's increased intracranial pressure following the elevation of the head of the bed. Mannitol 30 mg was administered intravenously based on the physician's orders. The patient's intracranial pressure began to decrease. It is important to note that the patient with TBI should never have the head of the bed elevated more than 30°. Quick evaluation and intervention may save your patient's life.

CLINICS CARE POINTS

Evidence-based-nursing implications include:

- Maintaining hemodynamic stability
- Monitoring for signs and symptoms of increased intracranial pressure
- Assessing coagulation panel, complete blood count, metabolic panel
- Symptom management
- Provision of psychosocial support

DISCLOSURE

The author has nothing to disclose.

REFERENCES

1. Ahmed S, Venigalla H, Mekala H, et al. Traumatic brain injury and neuropsychiatric complications. Indian psychiatric society; 2017. Available at: https://journals.sagepub.com/doi/pdf/10.4103/0253-7176.203129.
2. Centers for Disease Control. Traumatic brain injury and concussion. 2022. Available at: https://www.cdc.gov/traumaticbraininjury/index.html.
3. Boussard C, Holm L, Cancellier C, et al. Nonsurgical interventions after mild traumatic brain injury: a systematic review of results of the international collaboration on mild traumatic brain injury prognosis. Archives of physical medicine & rehabilitation 2014;95(3):S257–64.

4. Galgano M, Toshkezi G, Qiu X, et al. Traumatic brain injury. Cell 2017;26(7): 1118–30.

5. Hyder A, Wunderlich C, Puvanachandra P, et al. The impact of traumatic brain injuries: a global perspective. NeuroRehab 2007;22:341–53. Available at: https://content.iospress.com/download/neurorehabilitation/nre00374?id=neurorehabilitation%2Fnre00374.

6. Moppett I. Traumatic brain injury: assessment, resuscitation, and management. British journal of anesthesia 2007;99(1):18–31.

7. Czorlich P, Mader M, Emami P, et al. Operative versus non-operative treatment of traumatic brain injuries in patients 80 years and older. Neurosurg Rev 2020;43(5): 1305–14.

8. Damkliang J, Considine J, Kent B, et al. Using an evidence-based care bundle to improve initial emergency nursing management of patients with severe traumatic brain injury. J Clin Nurs 2015;24(23–24):3365–73.

9. Pujari R, Hutchinson P, Colius A. Surgical management of traumatic brain injury. Neurosurgical science 2018;62(5):584–92.

10. Modello S, Muller U, Jeromin A, et al. Blood-based diagnositics of traumatic brain injury. Expert molecular diagnostics 2011;11(1):65–78.

11. Varhese R, Chakrabarty J, Menon G. Nursing management of adults with severe traumatic brain injury: a narrative review. Indian J Crit Care Med 2017;21(10): 684–97.

The Complexity of Trauma for LGBTQ+ People
Considerations for Acute and Critical Care

Damon B. Cottrell, PhD, DNP, APRN, FNP-C, CCNS, ACNS-BC[a,b,]*,
Lori Aaron-Brija, DNP, APRN, FNP-C[c],
Emily Berkowitz, PhD, APRN, ANP-C, CVNP-BC, CNE[c],
Jeffrey Williams, DNP, APRN, CCNS[c]

KEYWORDS

- LGBT • LGBTQ+ • Trauma • Acute care • Welcoming environment

KEY POINTS

- Trauma care for lesbian, gay, bisexual, transgender, queer or questioning, and from other sexual and gender minority (LGBTQ+) patients is multifaceted and often includes emotional trauma.
- Anticipate the need for psychosocial support in LGBTQ+ patients who have experienced medical trauma.
- Be culturally aware of the LGBTQ+ population regarding specific needs and avoid compounding the trauma by implementing standards of care that are heteronormative in nature.
- Provide care by using a multidisciplinary and collaborative approach, assuring the best outcomes for LGBTQ+ patients who have experienced medical trauma.

INTRODUCTION

Trauma resulting in admission to acute or critical care has many sources. Trauma is categorized as blunt or penetrating mechanisms and burns. Some of the more common sources can include etiologies from motor vehicle collisions, falls, gunshot or stab wounds, and a myriad of others. In the acute and critical care setting, this is likely the most frequent context of trauma as a concept related to care. However, trauma care is much more complex.

[a] Texas Woman's University, PO Box 425498, ASB216N, Denton, TX 76204, USA; [b] Village Medical, 2774 E Eldorado Pkwy #100, Little Elm, TX 75068, USA; [c] Texas Woman's University, 5500 Southwestern Medical Avenue, Dallas, TX 75235, USA
* Correspondingauthor.
E-mail address: dcottrell@twu.edu

Crit Care Nurs Clin N Am 35 (2023) 179–189
https://doi.org/10.1016/j.cnc.2023.02.010
0899-5885/23/© 2023 Elsevier Inc. All rights reserved.

ccnursing.theclinics.com

Medical trauma is another facet that must be considered. Medical trauma ties the emotional and physical response to a traumatic event into a deeper understanding. Medical trauma can occur from an atraumatic sudden and life-threatening illness, complications from a medical procedure, an unexpected and worrisome diagnosis, constant noise, and sleep disruption, among others.[1]

The implications of trauma extend beyond our traditional thought. The health care experience for those who are lesbian, gay, bisexual, transgender (LGBT), queer or questioning, and from other sexual and gender minorities (LGBTQ+) is further complicated by their very being. Traumatic injury and medical trauma compounded the often lifetime experiences of trauma from stigma and discrimination. Clinicians must be aware of the complexity of trauma in acute and critical care settings to provide culturally appropriate care.

BACKGROUND

According to the US Census Bureau's Household Pulse Survey, an estimated 20 million people identify as LGBTQ+.[2] The report also suggests that 1% of the population is transgender, and half of the reported 8% of people identified as bisexual.[2] Recent estimates indicate an increase in the LGBTQ+ population; however, this is likely due to better opportunities to list sexual minorities or gender identity in survey instruments. Previous estimates of the LGBTQ+ population ranged from 3.5% in 2012 to 5.6% in 2020.[3] Considering the size of the population, it is probable that every health care provider has encountered people that identify within the LGBTQ+ community but may have been unaware of the patient's sexual orientation or gender identity.

The unexpected nature of traumatic injury does not always facilitate care that is LGBTQ+ appropriate, instead focusing on immediate pathology. However, this does not exempt trauma clinicians from learning about the LGBTQ+ community, and understanding the barriers, this population experiences. Clinician beliefs and biases regarding LGBTQ+ people are a significant barrier to providing skilled clinical and culturally competent care.[4] Previously held biases can affect how trauma care providers care for LGBTQ+ patients. This implicit bias is often automatic and frequently unintentional but does have the potential to influence decision-making.[5] Trauma care clinicians must acknowledge vulnerability to bias. This is an essential first step toward positive change.

HEALTH AND HEALTH CARE DISPARITY

One key to understanding the full scope of disparities in the LGBTQ+ population is related to the ability to collect identity data in large-scale surveys.[6] LGBTQ+ people have worse outcomes than heterosexual, cisgender people. Mental health disparities and poorer outcomes from chronic diseases such as obesity, asthma, arthritis, and cardiovascular disease are among the issues, along with higher rates of smoking, alcohol use, and many others.[7,8] Racial and socioeconomic variances also affect health outcomes and the ability to access care. Disparities start early. Compared with their heterosexual counterparts, LGBTQ+ people experience a disproportionately large number of adverse childhood events, including sexual abuse, emotional neglect, and abuse, physical abuse, living in a situation where mental illness is present in the household, among others.[9,10] Within the experiences of LGBTQ+ youth, these events are found to be higher in number and often result in worse outcomes over time.[10]

The health of LGBTQ+ people is theorized to be affected by discrimination, victimization, negative cultural values, beliefs, and stereotypes. The minority stress model has been used to research this for many years.[11] This model assumes that prejudice and social stress clearly play a role in untoward health outcomes.[12] Nurses should resist the perspective that being of a sexual and gender minority supposes poor outcomes and understand that the outcomes are from the harmful effects of stigma and discrimination.[7]

TRAUMA-RELATED ENTRY INTO ACUTE AND CRITICAL CARE

An unexpected traumatic event is the typical entry point into care. It also frequently begins with prehospital response and transport to acute care. There is a lack of research regarding aspects of care for LGBTQ+ patients who have experienced a need for transport to acute care settings. Within emergency department care, providers report difficulty with assessing patient histories from LGBTQ+ patients, particularly when their patients are transgendered. [13] Unfortunately, the same survey research indicated that there were witnessed discriminatory remarks made by providers and faculty members. Circumstances similar to those of heterosexual people may land LGBTQ+ patients into the acute and critical care setting. However, data reporting rates of intimate partner violence, suicidality, and violence including hate crimes, make the presence of an LGBTQ+ patient more complex.

Intimate Partner Violence

Intimate partner violence occurs when one member of a relationship commits physical or sexual violence on the other. This is distinguished from domestic violence, which can be carried out by any family member against another, such as parental abuse of a child.[14] The rates of intimate partner violence within the LGBTQ+ population as a whole are difficult to estimate due to a lack of research and suspected underreporting secondary to stigma and discrimination from both the health care and legal systems. Intimate partner violence is possibly more prevalent in LGBTQ+ couples than in heterosexual couples.[15] Intimate partner violence in aged LGBTQ+ patients has significant consequences, including a 300% increase in mortality and an increase in hospitalization.[16]

Suicidality

There are many factors thought to be associated with the higher rates of suicidality among LGBTQ+ persons, which are especially high among youth. The attempt of suicide may be as high as four times more likely in LGBTQ+ youth.[17,18] Up to 31% of LGBTQ+ persons report a lifetime suicide attempt, and most of them are made within 5 years of realization of sexual or gender minority status.[19] Overall, the rate of suicidality is 3 to 6 times greater in general among LGBTQ+ than for heterosexual, cisgender persons.[20] Methods differ between suicide attempts among LGBTQ+ and their heterosexual, cisgender counterparts. All subcategories studied in the National Violent Death Reporting System showed a preference for hanging/strangulation among LGBTQ+ persons, whereas firearms were preferred by heterosexual, cisgender males.[21] Only among lesbians was the use of firearms close to hanging in percentage of cases. The result of surviving an attempted hanging can range from severe hypoxic brain injury to full neurocognitive recovery depending on numerous factors such as time hanging, full cardiac arrest, and early intubation.[22]

Violence Victimization, Assault, and Hate Crime

Unfortunately, victimization begins early. The disparity in victimization of assault often starts in the school setting among adolescent LGBTQ+, who are twice as likely as their peers to be violently attacked before graduating high school.[23] Children and adolescents who identify as LGBTQ+ may experience physical dating violence and sexual dating violence, may be threatened or injured with a weapon while at school, bullied, and often feel unsafe when traveling to and while at school.[17,18] The prevalence of violence victimization was higher in transgender youth than in all other populations. [17]

The 2017 National Crime Victimization Survey found that LGBTQ+ people were three times more likely to be the victim of violent assault and even more likely to suffer serious injury.[24] Not only are members of this population more likely to be assaulted by those they know, but they are also victimized at high rates by strangers motivated by hate. Of hate crimes reported in 2020, 20% were based on sexual orientation, and 0.7% were based on gender identity.[25] Last year, 2021, was reported to be potentially the deadliest in America with regard to anti-trans motivated hate crime. [26] In the first half of 2022, there have been at least 26 transgender people killed.[27] Another consideration in all LGBTQ+-related stigma and discrimination is the potential presence of intersectionality. In the case of transgender people, transgender women of color experience exceptionally high rates of gender-motivated violence.[28]

NURSING CONSIDERATIONS

A significant first step to providing culturally appropriate and clinically relevant care for LGBTQ+ patients is to be informed. **Table 1** contains many definitions of the subpopulations of the LGBTQ+ population.[29] **Table 2** contains information about the differences between sex, gender, gender identity, and other highly relevant aspects of understanding those LGBTQ+.[30,31] Nurses should take the time to attend continuing education opportunities related to the experiences and care for those LGBTQ+ people. Then, inform others.

For clinicians who are unfamiliar with the care of transgender patients, it is essential to be interested but not curious. Learn about medical procedures that your patients may have undertaken and specifically how those procedures may alter the care. Gender-affirming surgeries include mastectomy or augmentation mammoplasty, often referred to as top surgery. They may have also had genital alterations such as penectomy, orchiectomy, and construction of a neovagina for trans women and total hysterectomy and phalloplasty for trans men, which are referred to as bottom surgery.[32] Trans women retain a prostate gland. Other procedures to feminize features include breast augmentation, vocal therapy, permanent hair removal, and throat and jawline surgeries.[33] For trans men who have had a neopenis constructed through phalloplasty, the trauma provider, should be aware that scarring and stricture of the newly lengthened urethra may cause an inability to pass a Foley catheter without causing traumatic damage and bleeding. Patients with potential for this complication should be treated with suprapubic catheter drainage until a dilation of the urethra can be safely accomplished.[34]

Less than 60% of transgender individuals have a primary care provider, which may lead to patients self-medicating by trial and error with unregulated, nonprescription hormone preparations ordered from overseas or bought illegally.[35] The lack of monitoring hormone levels, the potential for contamination, alteration, or substitution of the expected medications make this a risky manner of management.[36] For those patients who arrive in the critical care setting with no prescription records to guide dosages, this is a common difficulty.

Communication and Addressing Patients in the Context of Care

Nursing education and practice have a rich history of encouraging clinicians to develop cultural competence in dealing with special populations. It is essential to

Table 1 Commonly used LGBTQ+ terminology	
L—Lesbian	Female-identified person attracted romantically, erotically, and emotionally to other female-identified persons.
G—Gay	Someone who is emotionally, romantically, or sexually attracted to the same gender. Frequently refers to men attracted to men; however, women and nonbinary people may also use the term.
B—Bisexual	Individuals who are emotionally, romantically, and sexually attracted to people of their own gender and people of other sex or gender.
T—Transgendered	Term used for people who identify or express themselves differently from a cultural expectation or based on sex at birth. It does not imply sexual orientation.
Q—Queer	Queer connotes a multidimensional identity that often includes sexual orientations, gender identities, gender expressions, and sexual behaviors. Can also encompass cultural and political affiliations.
Q—Questioning	Questioning refers to people who are exploring their identity.
Other identities	
Asexual	Individuals who, within the spectrum of sexuality, may not experience sexual attraction to others.
Cisgender	Describes a person whose gender identity is aligned with sex at birth.
Gender-expansive	A person with a wide, flexible range of gender identity. May describe someone exploring their gender expression and/or gender identity.
Gender-fluid	A person who does not identify as a single gender.
Gender nonconforming	A broader term. Describes a person or people that do not act or behaving in a way that fits with traditional expectations of gender.
Gender-queer	Describes a person or people that embrace fluidity of gender.
Intersex	Individuals born with naturally occurring variations of chromosomes, hormones, genitalia, and other sex characteristics. It may be impossible to determine the genetic gender of the client without karyotyping.
Nonbinary	Describes a person who doesn't identify as a man or a woman. This could refer to both, or something outside of a male or female category.
Pansexual	Individuals whose attractions, whether emotional or sexual are not limited by biological sex or gender.
Same-gender Loving	May be a preferred term for those who are lesbian, gay, or bisexual.

Adapted from Human Rights Campaign. Glossary of terms. Human Rights Campaign Web site. https://www.hrc.org/resources/glossary-of-terms. Updated n.d. Accessed Aug 28, 2022.

understand the complexity of the issues surrounding culturally competent care of patients who are LGBTQ+ when the sociopolitical environment encourages nondisclosure of sexual orientation or gender identity. Unless, and possibly even if, the clinician is of a sexual or gender minority, a shift toward cultural humility is encouraged. Instead, the difference implies the competence of the nurse as an expert, whereas cultural humility respects the patient as the expert.[37]

The manner in which we address our patients and families is key. Best practices include using the name and pronouns preferred by the patient rather than relying on legal documentation alone.[32] Pronouns can be gender binary, such as she/her/hers or he/him/his or may be gender neutral. Gender neutral pronouns may include ze/

Table 2	
Delineation between sex and gender	
Sex	Refers to sex assigned at birth, that is, male or female. Usually based on the appearance of external genitalia.
Sexual orientation	Refers to a person's emotional, romantic, and/or sexual attraction to men, women, neither, or both.
Gender	A personal identity. A construct.
Gender identity	Refers to an innermost concept of self as male, female, both, or neither.
Gender expression	Refers to external appearance, how a person expresses externally. May or may not conform to social norms.

Adapted from Acquaviva K. Improving the critical care experience of LGBTQ patients and families. Society of Critical Care Medicine (SCCM) Web site. https://sccm.org/Communications/Critical-Connections/Archives/2017/Improving-the-Critical-Care-Experience-of-LGBTQ-Pa. Updated 2017. Accessed Aug 20, 2022; Human Rights Campaign. Glossary of terms. Human Rights Campaign Web site. https://www.hrc.org/resources/glossary-of-terms. Updated n.d. Accessed Aug 28, 2022; and White T, Smith J. Sex versus gender: What's the difference and why does it matter? Psych Central Web site. https://psychcentral.com/health/sex-vs-gender. Updated 2022. Accessed Aug 28, 2022.

hir/hirs, ze/zir/zirs, Xe/Xem/Xyr, or others may prefer them/their/theirs. When unsure of which pronoun to use for a patient, it is commonly acceptable to use the more generic pronoun "they" or a last name, as in patient Jones, until you can ask the patient what pronoun they prefer.

To provide a safe and healing environment, all members of the health care team should be aware of the patient's preferred name and gender pronouns. If the legal name and gender do not match the patient's preferences, it is important to explain to the patient that for the purposes of medication administration and testing, they will be asked to confirm the name that is on their legal identification. Most patients will understand and are often quite forgiving of this nuance in care. Because more than 60% of transgender patients have not changed their legal identification documents to match their lived experience, this is a common situation for clinicians to encounter; however, it is important to affirm recognition with the patient of their preferences.[38] Key recommendations for clinicians include approaching transgender patients with sensitivity and awareness of barriers to trusting relationships due to prior negative health care experiences, maintaining open communication with the promise of confidentiality for the patient, and using gender-inclusive language such as "partner" instead of "girl/boyfriend."[33]

Several strategies may help with communication in acute care settings. A simple one could allow employees the option of displaying their preferred pronouns on their employee badges. A conversation with every conscious, communicative patient about their wishes for decision-making is necessary. Nurses should address advance directives and assist in completing one if necessary. Seven questions are recommended for all conscious and communicative patients, whereas in acute care, these are found in **Box 1**.[30] This approach provides a solid foundation for building trust in the provision of care.

Acute care organizations should update admission assessment forms and all references to sex and gender within the electronic health record. Evidence suggests that this is becoming more the norm and has momentum toward appropriate and inclusive language that allows for more than just the binary sex system.[39] Electronic health record prompts can be used to guide information gathering in a nonjudgmental manner, allowing LGBTQ+ patients to feel included. It is important to understand that the data

> **Box 1**
> **Helpful patient intake questions**
>
> What name would you like to be called?
>
> What sex were you assigned at birth?
>
> What gender do you identify as?
>
> What pronouns would you prefer us to use when we refer to you?
>
> Who are the people you consider to be family?
>
> What information can we share with your family about your illness, condition, injury, or care?
>
> What information would you not like us to share with them?
>
> *Adapted from* Acquaviva K. Improving the critical care experience of LGBTQ patients and families. Society of Critical Care Medicine (SCCM) Web site. https://sccm.org/Communications/Critical-Connections/Archives/2017/Improving-the-Critical-Care-Experience-of-LGBTQ-Pa. Updated 2017. Accessed Aug 20, 2022.

collected are visible to every provider involved in the care of the LGBT+ client, assuring that all the providers and staff are aware of the client's gender identity.

Creating a Welcoming Environment

Health care facilities should create a welcoming and inclusive environment for those in the LGBTQ+ community by making the setting comfortable and safe. However, the amount of research on this topic that pertains to the acute care setting is limited. The thought and strategies for creating a welcoming environment for LGBTQ+ patients can be used and perhaps modified within the acute care setting. One strategy is the placement of LGBTQ+ focused reading materials in waiting rooms and lobbies, such as educational pamphlets on testing for sexually transmitted infections, intimate partner violence and resources for support services. Waiting room walls can also display the faces of the LGBTQ+ community.[39] Hospitals can also provide visual cues signifying everyone is welcome by posting the facility's nondiscrimination statement. Acute organizations can help create a welcoming environment with gender-neutral restrooms. Existing restrooms can be simply modified by adding locks to doors.

Implementing Trauma-Informed Care

Trauma-informed care, a specialized approach for a person who has experienced trauma, is pertinent for LGBTQ+ patients. LGBTQ+ patients often feel marginalized by society and discriminated against in interactions with the health care system.[9] The disproportionately high rates of trauma experienced by LBGTQ+ individuals make developing a trusting relationship with health care providers a challenge. Distrust of the health care environment and health care providers is present in up to 73% of transgender people and up to 23% of lesbian, gay, or bisexual people.[40] Within the schema of trauma-informed care, three components of trauma are to be considered, including events, experiences, and effects.[41] The principles of trauma-informed care are to ensure safety; foster trustworthiness and transparency; provide peer support; engage in collaboration and mutuality; empower patients; and understand the cultural, historical, and gender issues that may be grounded in the experience.[41]

SUMMARY

Trauma care is complex. Care focused on the injury or event is compounded by the need to establish an environment of psychological safety for the LGBTQ+ patient. This begins with establishing a baseline of respect and assurance of dignity in the provision of care. Recognizing the impact of traumatic stress on critical care patients as it affects their ability to cope with the stresses of treatment is vital, and simple actions can help to decrease discomfort. Acute and critical care clinicians have a significant opportunity to effect great change outside of the physical recovery of a trauma patient. This can have new meaning to our healing environments. When it is apparent to a patient that the providers caring for them are comfortable working with LGBTQ+ clients, stress can be minimized and healing optimized. We have significant opportunities to mitigate many of the barriers that are encountered by the LGBTQ+ community within health care.

CLINICS CARE POINTS

- Use appropriate language and terminology when addressing LGBTQ+ patients.
- Be sure to screen for intimate partner violence, violent crime causality, and suicidality.
- Consistently use trauma-informed strategies when providing care.

REFERENCES

1. International society for traumatic stress studies. What is medical trauma?. 2020. Available at: https://istss.org/ISTSS_Main/media/Documents/Public-Facing-Fact-Sheet-2.pdf. Accessed August 20, 2022.
2. Powell L. We are here: understanding the size of the LGBTQ+ community. 2021. https://www.hrc.org/press-releases/we-are-here-lgbtq-adult-population-in-united-states-reaches-at-least-20-million-according-to-human-rights-campaign-foundation-report.
3. Jones J. LGBT identification rises to 5.6% in the latest U.S. estimate. Gallup.com Web site. 2021. Available at: https://news.gallup.com/poll/329708/lgbt-identification-rises-latest-estimate.aspx.
4. Kaiafas K, Kennedy T. Lesbian, gay, bisexual, transgender, queer cultural competency training to improve the quality of care: an evidence-based practice project. J Emerg Nurs 2021;47(4):654–60.
5. Ruhl C. Implicit or unconscious bias. 2020. Available at: https://www.simplypsychology.org/. https://www.simplypsychology.org/implicit-bias.html. Accessed July 9, 2022.
6. Cahill S, Makadon H. Sexual orientation and gender identity data collection in clinical settings and in electronic health records: a key to ending LGBT health disparities. LGBT Health 2014;1(1).
7. Valdiserri R, Holtgrave D, Poteat T, et al. Unraveling health disparities among sexual and gender minorities: a commentary on the persistent impact of stigma. J homosexuality 2019;66(5):571–89. Available at: https://www.tandfonline.com/doi/abs/10.1080/00918369.2017.1422944.
8. Medina-Martínez J, Saus-Ortega C, Sánchez-Lorente MM, et al. Health inequities in LGBT people and nursing interventions to reduce them: a systematic review.

Int J Environ Res Public Health 2021;18(22). Available at: https://search.proquest.com/docview/2602065582.

9. Levenson J, Craig S, Austin. Trauma-informed and affirmative mental health practices with LGBTQ+ clients. Psychol Serv 2023;20(Suppl 1):134–44.

10. Craig S, Austin A, Levenson J, et al. Frequencies and patterns of adverse childhood events in LGBTQ+ youth. Child Abuse Neglect 2020;107:104623.

11. Hoy-Ellis C. Minority stress and mental health: a review of the literature. J Homosexuality 2021. ahead-of-print(ahead-of-print):1-25 Available at: https://www.tandfonline.com/doi/abs/10.1080/00918369.2021.2004794.

12. Meyer I. Prejudice, social stress, and mental health in lesbian, gay, and bisexual populations. Psychol Sex orientation Gend Divers 2013;1(S):3–26. Available at: https://search.proquest.com/docview/1419378860.

13. Moll J, Krieger P, Heron S, et al. Attitudes, behavior, and comfort of emergency medicine residents in caring for LGBT patients: what do we know? AEM Educ Train 2019;3(2):129–35. Available at: https://onlinelibrary.wiley.com/doi/abs/10.1002/aet2.10318.

14. Mims D, Waddell R. An examination of intimate partner violence and sexual violence among individuals who identify as lesbian, gay, bi-sexual, and/or transgender (LBGTQ). Environ Soc Psychol 2021;6.

15. Rollè L, Giardina G, Caldarera A, et al. When intimate partner violence meets same sex couples: a review of same sex intimate partner violence. Front Psychol 2018;9:1506. Available at: https://www.ncbi.nlm.nih.gov/pubmed/30186202.

16. Hillman J. Intimate partner violence among older LGBT adults: unique risk factors, issues in reporting and treatment, and recommendations for research, practice, and policy. In: Russell B, editor. Intimate partner violence and the LGBT+ community. Springer; 2020.

17. Johns M, Lowry R, Andrzejewski J, et al. Transgender identity and experiences of violence victimization, substance use, suicide risk, and sexual risk behaviors among high school students — 19 states and large urban school districts, 2017. MMWR Morb Mortal Wkly Rep 2019;68(3):67–71. Available at: https://www.cdc.gov/mmwr/volumes/68/wr/mm6803a3.htm. Accessed Aug 27, 2022.

18. Johns M, Lowry R, Haderxhanaj L, et al. Trends in violence victimization and suicide risk by sexual identity among high school students — youth risk behavior survey, United States, 2015–2019. MMWR Suppl 2020;69(1):19–27. Available at: https://www.cdc.gov/mmwr/volumes/69/su/su6901a3.htm. Accessed Aug 27, 2022.

19. Meyer I, Blosnich J, Choi S, et al. Suicidal behavior and coming out milestones in three cohorts of sexual minority adults. LGBT health 2021;8(5):34–348. Available at: https://www.liebertpub.com/doi/abs/10.1089/lgbt.2020.0466.

20. Ramchand R, Schuler M, Schoenbaum M, et al. Suicidality among sexual minority adults: gender, age, and race/ethnicity differences. Am J Prev Med 2022;62(2):193–202.

21. Lyons BH, Walters ML, Jack SPD, et al. Suicides among lesbian and gay male individuals: findings from the national violent death reporting system. Am J Prev Med 2019;56(4):512–21. Available at: https://www.sciencedirect.com/science/article/pii/S074937971832436X.

22. de Charentenay L, Schnell G, Pichon N, et al. Outcomes in 886 critically ill patients after near-hanging injury. Chest 2020;158(6):2404–13. Available at: https://www.sciencedirect.com/science/article/pii/S0012369220320912.

23. De Pedro K, Lynch R, Esqueda M. Understanding safety, victimization and school climate among rural lesbian, gay, bisexual, transgender, and questioning

(LGBTQ) youth. J LGBT youth 2018;15(4):265–79. Available at: https://www.tandfonline.com/doi/abs/10.1080/19361653.2018.1472050.

24. Flores AR, Haider-Markel DP, Lewis DC, et al. Antidiscrimination interventions, political ads on transgender rights, and public opinion: results from two survey experiments on adults in the United States. Front Psychol 2021;12:729322. Available at: https://search.proquest.com/docview/2570114400.

25. United States Department of Justice. 2020 hate crime statistics: FBI releases 2020 hate crime statistics. United States Department of Justice Web site. Available at: https://www.justice.gov/hatecrimes/hate-crime-statistics. Accessed August 20, 2022.

26. Natividad I. Why is anti-trans violence on the rise in America? Berkeley News 2021. Available at: https://news.berkeley.edu/2021/06/25/why-is-anti-trans-violence-on-the-rise-in-america/.

27. HRC Foundation. Fatal violence against the transgender and gender non-conforming community in 2022. Human Rights Campaign Web site. 2022. Available at: https://www.hrc.org/resources/fatal-violence-against-the-transgender-and-gender-non-conforming-community-in-2022. Accessed Aug 28, 2022.

28. Gyamerah A, Baguso G, Santiago-Rodriguez E, et al. Experiences and factors associated with transphobic hate crimes among transgender women in the san francisco bay area: comparisons across race. BMC public health 2021;21(1):1–1053. Available at: https://search.proquest.com/docview/2543504791.

29. Human Rights Campaign. Glossary of terms. Human rights Campaign Web site. Available at: https://www.hrc.org/resources/glossary-of-terms. Accessed August 28, 2022.

30. Acquaviva K. Improving the critical care experience of LGBTQ patients and families. Society of Critical Care Medicine (SCCM) Web site. 2017. Available at: https://sccm.org/Communications/Critical-Connections/Archives/2017/Improving-the-Critical-Care-Experience-of-LGBTQ-Pa. Accessed August 20, 2022.

31. White T, Smith J. Sex vs. gender: what's the difference and why does it matter? Psych Central Web site. 2022. https://psychcentral.com/health/sex-vs-gender. Accessed August 28, 2022.

32. Rosendale N, Goldman S, Ortiz G, et al. Acute clinical care for transgender patients: a review. JAMA Intern Med 2018;178(11):1535–43. Available at: https://search.ebscohost.com/login.aspx?direct=true&db=mnh&AN=30178031&site=ehost-live.

33. Klein DA, Paradise SL, Goodwin ET. Caring for transgender and gender-diverse persons: what clinicians should know. Am Fam Physician 2018;98(11):645–53.

34. Davis W, Patel B, Thurmond J. Emergency care considerations for the transgender patient: complications of gender-affirming treatments. J Emerg Nurs 2021;47(1):33–9. Available at: https://search.ebscohost.com/login.aspx?direct=true&db=cmedm&AN=33023789&site=ehost-live.

35. Abeln B, Love R. Considerations for the care of transgender individuals. Nurs Clin North Am 2019;54(4):551–9. Available at: https://search.ebscohost.com/login.aspx?direct=true&db=mnh&AN=31703780&site=ehost-live.

36. Joseph A, Cliffe C, Hillyard M, et al. Gender identity and the management of the transgender patient: a guide for non-specialists. J R Soc Med 2017;110(4):144–52. Available at: https://search.ebscohost.com/login.aspx?direct=true&db=cmedm&AN=28382847&site=ehost-live.

37. Ruud M. Cultural humility in the care of individuals who are lesbian, gay, bisexual, transgender, or queer. Nursing For Womens Health 2018;22(3):255–63. https://doi.org/10.1016/j.nwh.2018.03.009.
38. Goldhammer H, Malina S, Keuroghlian A. Communicating with patients who have nonbinary gender identities. Ann Fam Med 2018;16(6):559–62. Available at: https://www.clinicalkey.es/playcontent/1-s2.0-S1544170919300666.
39. Menkin D, Tice D, Flores D. Implementing inclusive strategies to deliver high-quality LGBTQ+ care in health care systems. J Nurs Manage 2020;30(5): O46–51.
40. Human Rights Campaign. Healthcare equality index 2022. Human rights campaign. 2022. Available at: https://reports.hrc.org/hei-2022. Accessed August 28, 2022.
41. Substance Abuse and Mental Health Services Administration. SAMHSA's concept of trauma and guidance for a trauma-informed approach. Substance Abuse Ment Health Serv Adm 2014.

Management of Intra-abdominal Traumatic Injury

Shannon S. Gaasch, MS, CRNP, AGACNP-BC[1],*,
Christopher L. Kolokythas, MS, AGACNP-BC, ACCNS-AG, CRNP, APRN-CNS[1]

KEYWORDS

- Trauma • Resuscitation • Coagulopathy • Hemorrhage • Abdominal • Injury
- Laparotomy • Penetrating

KEY POINTS

- Permissive hypotension, reversal of coagulopathy, and balanced transfusion strategy are important during the resuscitation phase.
- If the patient is hemodynamically unstable and unable to receive a computed tomography scan to evaluate injuries, the patient should be immediately taken to the operating room.
- Perform routine physical examinations, ultrasound imaging, and laboratory data to ensure patient's stability.
- Early transfusion and limiting crystalloid administration are recommended.

Traumatic injuries occur from unintentional and intentional violent events, claiming an estimated 4.4 million lives annually.[1] Abdominal trauma accounts for roughly 15% of all trauma-related hospitalizations.[2] Abdominal trauma can be subcategorized into blunt or penetrating, with blunt abdominal trauma (BAT) being more prevalent.[3] Penetrating abdominal trauma (PAT) occurs when the abdominal cavity is breached by an external object that penetrates the tissue at variable velocities.[4] Understanding the impact mechanism, amount of force, and anatomic trajectory assists in developing a focused clinical evaluation. Additionally, the anatomic location of the impact site along with entrance and exit wounds gives the clinician clues as to which organ systems are of primary concern: peritoneal, retroperitoneal, or pelvic. The extent of the injury depends on the velocity, the transfer of energy from the projectile to the tissues (dependent on caliber size, shape, and design), and the elasticity of the affected tissues.[5]

MECHANISMS AND INJURY PATTERNS

The most common causes of BAT are related to automobile and motorcycle crashes, pedestrian–automobile collisions, falls, assaults, and industrial accidents.[2,6] Injuries

University of Maryland Medical Center, R Adams Cowley Shock Trauma Center, USA
[1] Present address: 22 South Greene Street, Baltimore MD 21201
* Corresponding author. 22 South Greene Street, Baltimore, MD 21201.
E-mail address: shannon.gaasch@umm.edu

Crit Care Nurs Clin N Am 35 (2023) 191–211
https://doi.org/10.1016/j.cnc.2023.02.011
ccnursing.theclinics.com

result from a combination of crushing, deforming, stretching, and shearing forces that can cause variable acceleration and deceleration patterns depending on the direction of impact.[6] Injuries to the spleen, liver, and small bowel are most common with BAT as a result of the external compression of the abdominal viscera against the posterior body structures.[7] The force of injury can damage the parenchyma of solid organs as well as rupture the vasculature, causing organ contusion and intra-abdominal hemorrhage. Anterior BAT typically affects the liver, spleen, pancreas, major blood vessels, and gut. Posterior trauma typically affects the kidneys and spine.[7]

The incidence of hospitalization from PAT in urban trauma centers is about 35% and 12% in rural settings.[8] Common mechanisms of injury include stabbings, gun violence, industrial incidents, and explosive injuries.[9] Penetrating abdominal stab wounds typically involve the liver, small bowel, diaphragm, and colon.[7] In shallow posterior penetrations such as a stab wound, deep organs are buffered by large muscle groups in the back.[7] A bullet can cause injury to anything in its pathway.[10] It is critical to understand the anatomy to be able to determine potential injury from the bullet trajectory. The most commonly injured abdominal organs from gunshots are the small and large bowel, liver, and intra-abdominal vasculature.[10] High velocity, high energy transfer injuries of penetrating trauma are associated with an eightfold increase in mortality rates compared with injuries related to low velocity, low energy transfer stab wounds[3] (Table 1).

Hemorrhage control is a top priority in trauma management, as it is the leading contributor to death and is the most preventable cause of death in trauma.[11] Traumatic abdominal injuries have significant morbidity and mortality rates, however, patients who are hemodynamically stable can usually be observed without surgical intervention.[7]

EVALUATION, ASSESSMENT, AND DIAGNOSIS

On initial presentation, the Advanced Trauma Life Support (ATLS) primary survey should be followed in sequential order to identify life-threatening conditions (Box 1).[7] A detailed history should be obtained when possible as it may guide potential management.[10] Abdominal trauma can be challenging to assess as the damage is usually internal. The abdominal cavity can hold a significant amount of blood without a change in size, appearance, or peritoneal irritation, which can delay diagnosis of injury and increase morbidity and mortality.[7] Additionally, assessment and diagnosis can be confounded by poor history, distracting injuries, and altered mental status.[4] Abdominal examination alone does not reliably classify or differentiate patients with intra-abdominal injuries.[6] A thorough physical assessment in conjunction with other diagnostics can provide guidance in deciding to manage the patient conservatively,

Table 1 Common injuries in abdominal trauma[3]		
	Blunt Injury	**Penetrating Injury**
Mechanism	Crushing, deforming, stretching, and shearing forces	• Breach of the peritoneal cavity from ballistic or non-ballistic trauma (stabs, bone fragments) • Ballistic trauma creates primary and secondary blast effect
Common Injuries	Spleen and liver	• Large bowel • Small bowel • Intra-abdominal vasculature

---

Box 1
Key principles of primary survey[7]

Airway maintenance with restriction of cervical spine motion	• Ensure airway patency, assess for any foreign bodies or injuries that may cause obstruction
	• Placement of advanced (endotracheal tube or tracheostomy) airway should not be delayed
	• If the GCS is ≤ 8 then an advanced airway should be placed
	• Reevaluation of airway patency should be done periodically
Breathing and ventilation	• Airway patency does not ensure adequate ventilation
	• Oxygen should be applied and monitor pulse oximetry
	• Expose patient's chest to evaluate tracheal position, chest wall excursion, and jugular vein distention
	• Assess for signs of hemothorax, pneumothorax, tension pneumothorax, or tracheal or bronchial injuries
Circulation with hemorrhage control	• Controlling hemorrhage is crucial
	• Once tension pneumothorax is ruled out, assume hypotension is due to hemorrhage
	• Aggressive fluid resuscitation is not a substitute for hemorrhage control
	• Fluid resuscitation with 1L crystalloid, if not responsive then initiate colloid resuscitation
	• Clinical assessments of level of consciousness, skin perfusion, and pulse can provide information about the patient's intravascular volume status
	• Altered level of consciousness, ashen gray facial skin and pale extremities and/or a rapid thready pulse are signs of hypovolemia
Disability (assessment of neurologic status)	• Evaluation of level of consciousness, pupillary size and reaction, and evidence of lateralizing signs (and if present determine what spinal cord level)
Exposure/Environment	• Expose patient completely to assess for wounds and injuries, then keep patient covered with blankets and external warming devices
	• If hypothermia is present on admission be sure to correct it rapidly as hypothermia can exacerbate hemorrhage.

---

with angiography, or with surgery. In a hemodynamically unstable patient, surgical exploration may be required before imaging is obtained.[7] Signs of peritonitis, abdominal distention, nausea, vomiting, low urine output, ecchymosis, bleeding from rectum, and tenderness to palpation may be present on examination and could suggest potential injury.

The use of imaging techniques aids in assessing injury and the development of a management plan. Focused Assessment with Sonography for Trauma (FAST) examination, computed tomography (CT), and x-ray can be used non-invasively for diagnosis and characterization of injury severity and trajectory.[8] The FAST examination includes ultrasound evaluation of the pericardial sac, hepatorenal fossa, splenorenal fossa, and pelvis or pouch of Douglas. This can be used to diagnose pericardial effusion, peritoneal, retroperitoneal, and pelvic bleeding. The FAST has limited sensitivity in diagnosing hollow viscus injury or any injury with the presence of subcutaneous emphysema. Additionally, body habitus and user experience can affect the quality and interpretation of the study[7] (**Fig. 1**).[12]

Direct peritoneal lavage (DPL) is an additional study that can be quickly performed to diagnose the presence of bowel perforation or intra-abdominal bleeding from BAT. After gastric and urinary decompression, a needle is inserted into the peritoneal cavity and a saline lavage is instilled and aspirated, showing possible blood or enteric contamination. This technique is easily performed but is used less frequently with the rise in ultrasound use and the prevalence of the less invasive FAST examination[13] (**Fig. 2**).

PHYSIOLOGIC IMPACT AND RESUSCITATION RECOMMENDATION

The presentation of a patient with PAT or BAT may reveal shock, hypotension, tachypnea, and signs of end-organ perfusion dysfunction (oliguria, cool and mottled extremities, elevated lactate).[14] Unstable patients with abdominal trauma typically require surgical intervention, and penetrating injuries prompt an exploratory laparotomy if there is hemodynamic instability, the presence of entrance and exit wounds, peritoneal irritation, or evisceration.[7]

One common misconception in the acute care setting is that vital signs alone can be relied on to diagnose hypovolemia; however, vital signs can be affected by numerous clinical conditions.[15,16] Severe shock may be present with "normal vital signs" as compensatory mechanisms will transiently maintain blood pressure in the face of profound metabolic acidosis.[7,17] Some patients, particularly young healthy patients, are able to compensate until they have reached stage III of shock, necessitating the use of alternative assessment techniques[7] (**Box 2**). Oftentimes, multiple assessment modalities are being used simultaneously by the care team (eg, bedside ultrasound, physical examination, hemodynamic monitoring).

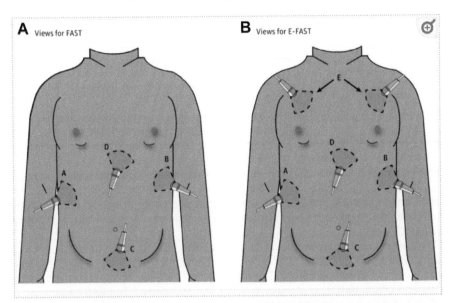

Fig. 1. FAST views. (*From* Kornblith AE, Addo N, Plasencia M, et al. Development of a Consensus-Based Definition of Focused Assessment With Sonography for Trauma in Children. JAMA Netw Open. 2022;5(3):e222922. Published 2022 Mar 1. doi:10.1001/jamanetworkopen.2022.2922 (Kornblith).)

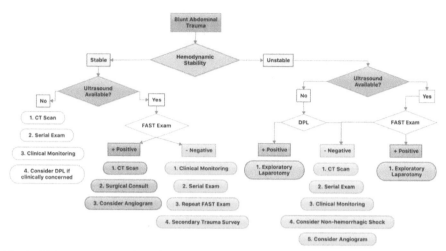

Fig. 2. BAT management algorithm.

Complex physiologic derangements occur after traumatic injury and prompt recognition and control of hemorrhage are critical to prevent systemic effects.[18] Direct tissue injury generates a local response, propagating a systemic reaction that can be significantly amplified and harmful. Three key factors should be addressed for trauma patients, hypothermia, trauma-induced coagulopathy (TIC), and acidosis, known as the lethal triad (**Fig. 3**).[19] **Table 2** demonstrates the clinical significance, physiologic effect, and treatment recommendations for each key factor.

Box 2
Modalities to assess hemodynamic status[7,16]

Non-invasive monitoring (BP)
  Limited reliability in severe hypovolemic shock
  Inaccurate in marked shock due to severe peripheral vasoconstriction[17]

Invasive monitoring (arterial line, central venous pressure, pulmonary artery catheter, and so on)

DPL
  Invasive procedure, requires surgical expertise, quickly identifies intra-abdominal injury
  Non-repeatable and can interfere with interpretation of the CT scan or FAST examination[7]
  CT scan and FAST are preferred assessment modalities, if not available, DPL is then performed

Passive leg raise
  If a 10% - 12% increase in cardiac output is observed with the maneuver then the patient is likely a fluid responder[16]

Pulse oximetry
  Limited use in acute management of shock
  Helpful in the post-resuscitation period to ensure appropriate peripheral tissue perfusion[17]

Bedside ultrasonography
  Measuring inferior vena cava collapsibility and velocity time integral to estimate intravascular volume status and determine need for further resuscitation[16]
  FAST can rule out hemoperitoneum, hemopericardium, tamponade physiology, and pneumothorax or hemothorax (see **Fig. 1**).

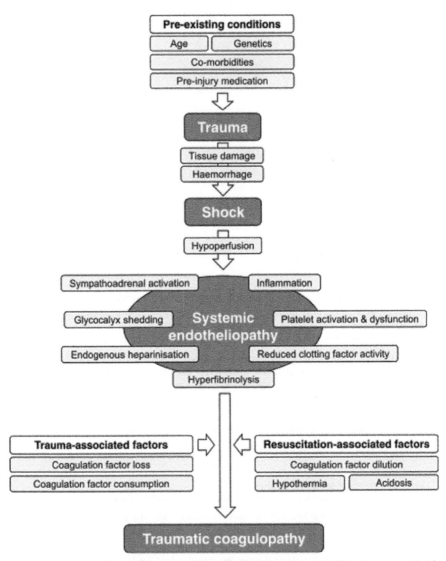

Fig. 3. TIC reprinted from Open Access from Spahn, Donat R., et al. "The European Guideline on Management of Major Bleeding and Coagulopathy Following Trauma: Fifth Edition." *Critical Care*, vol. 23, no. 1, 27 Mar. 2019, pp. 2347–3., doi.org/10.1186/s13054-019-2347-3.

Laboratory results in conjunction with invasive hemodynamic monitoring and physical assessment will guide resuscitation (**Box 3**).[20] Lactate and base deficit are markers of anaerobic metabolism and should be trended to track the recovery from shock at the cellular level.[20] Persistent metabolic acidosis indicates ongoing blood loss or inadequate resuscitation and volume resuscitation is the standard of care. Sodium bicarbonate should not be administered to treat hypovolemic shock.[7] If ongoing blood loss is suspected, a surgeon should be notified to assess the need for re-exploration or angioembolization.

Table 2
Key factors of lethal triad of trauma[20-23]

	Clinical Features/Significance	Physiologic Effect	Prevention/Treatment
Hypothermia	• Core body temperature <35°C[20] • Occurs from physical exposure, intoxication, circulatory changes, and cold fluids[21]	• Has profound effect on coagulation factors (reduces factor activity by 10% for every degree decrease in temperature)[20,21] • Severity of hypothermia associated with increased mortality rate, 70%–100% in severe hypothermia	• Maintain core body temperature > 35 C • Minimize exposure with convection blankets, warmed fluids, decreasing operating room time • Controlling hemorrhage is important for correcting hypothermia[20]
Coagulopathy	• 30% of trauma patients present with TIC • Poor outcomes associated with inflammatory mediators released from tissue injury and secondary tissue hypoxia[22]	• TIC begins 30 min after injury; clotting cascade activated after injury, clot is formed and depletes platelets and coagulation factors leading to a consumptive coagulopathy • Worsens with fluid administration and red blood cells (no clotting factor administration[22] • Fibrinolysis is a key feature of TIC, occurring within the first hour after trauma and is associated with mortality rates as high as 90%[23]	• Transfuse clotting factors early, use 1:1:1 transfusion strategy[22] • Limit excessive crystalloid administration
Acidosis	• Hemorrhage causes decreased circulatory volume and delivery of oxygen to tissues. • Toxic metabolites, anaerobic metabolism and lactic acidosis develop. • Degree of acidosis and lactate levels on admission predict mortality in trauma patients[20]	• When pH homeostasis is disrupted, enzymatic function throughout the body occurs and multiple organ dysfunction (MOD) develops • Decreased cardiac contractility and cardiac output, vasodilation, hypotension, and bradycardia are seen in MOD.[22]	• Optimize oxygen delivery through blood transfusions and cardiac output augmentation with pharmacologic agents while controlling hemorrhage to prevent significant acidosis[17,20]

Box 3
Box 3 **Laboratory data to collect[20]**
ABG
CBC
CMP
INR
PT
PTT
TEG or ROTEM
Fibrinogen
Myoglobin
Lactate
Abbreviations: ABG, arterial blood gas; CBC, complete blood count; CMP, complete metabolic panel; INR, international normalized ratio; PT, prothrombin time; PTT, partial thrombin time; ROTEM, rotational thromboelastometry; TEG, thromboelastography.

Damage Control Surgery

Defined as the planned temporary sacrifice of normal anatomy to preserve physiologic function, Damage Control Surgery (DCS) focuses on the management of abdominal bleeding through surgical suture, ligation, or cauterization.[23,24] During DCS, the goal is not for primary repair of injuries, but instead for control of hemorrhage and peritoneal contamination with the use of peritoneal packing and temporary closure to restore homeostasis. Attention should be directed to metabolic derangements rather than definitive control. This method revolutionized trauma care and drastically reduced mortality related to hemorrhage.[23]

Damage Control Resuscitation

The objective of Damage Control Resuscitation (DCR) is restoring homeostasis in the actively bleeding patient by preventing or mitigating tissue hypoxia, oxygen debt, and coagulopathy.[23] The core principles of DCR include permissive hypotension, fluid restriction, and fixed-ratio transfusion strategies (**Fig. 4**).[19,23] Allowing for permissive hypotension aims to target the minimum blood pressure (BP) necessary to perfuse organs. Targeting a normal BP can displace clots formed during the body's attempt at hemostasis, lead to over-resuscitation, increased bleeding related to dilutional coagulopathy (DC), and exacerbation of tissue hypoxia.[23] Specific BP targets have yet to be defined, but current data suggest a systolic BP (SBP) of 80 to 100 mm Hg. An SBP target of >100 mm Hg is recommended for patients with traumatic brain injury (TBI), patients 50 to 69 year old, and an SBP >110 mm Hg for those with TBI younger than 49 year old.[19] A normal BP should be targeted once hemostasis has been obtained.

Aggressive fluid resuscitation in a patient actively hemorrhaging can contribute to more bleeding and DC.[23] Higher crystalloid-to-packed red blood cell (PRBC) transfusion ratios have been associated with a 70% increased risk of multiple organ failure and are twice as likely to lead to acute respiratory distress syndrome and abdominal compartment syndrome.[19] A more balanced approach to fluid resuscitation is

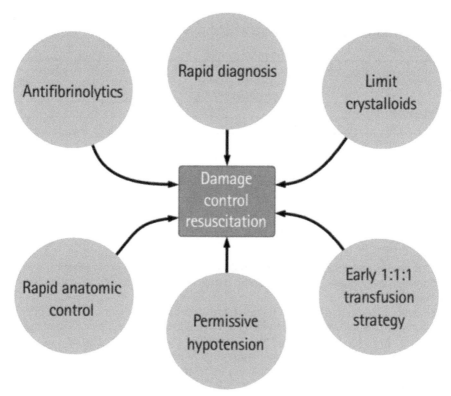

Fig. 4. Principles of DCR. *From* Evan Leibner et al. "Damage control resuscitation." Clinical and experimental emergency medicine, vol. 7, no. 1 (2020): 5-13. doi:10.15441/ceem.19.089.

recommended by the ATLS guidelines, with a maximum transfusion of 1 to 2 L of crystalloid and early transfusion of blood products.[7]

The separation of whole blood into blood components has led to greater administration of PRBCs versus plasma and platelets during resuscitation efforts, contributing to DC and other complications for the severely injured. Balanced transfusion is the administration of blood products in a ratio more equivalent to that of whole blood: 1 PRBC to 1 plasma to 1 platelet to 1 cryoprecipitate unit. Compared with crystalloid resuscitation, balanced product transfusion resolves acidosis, prevents endothelial damage, treats TIC, and begins to reverse DC.[22] Transfusing platelets and plasma early in the balanced transfusion strategy has also been associated with improved survival following trauma.[7] If available, TEG or rotational thromboelastometry (should) be used along with PT, PTT, INR, and fibrinogen to help guide blood product resuscitation and identify clotting deficiencies.[7] Administration of tranexamic acid (TXA) could be considered for the severely injured patient with uncontrollable hemorrhage or fibrinolysis to aid the development of a stronger clot.[7] TXA has been shown to decrease mortality when administered within 1 to 3 hours after injury.[7,25] The therapeutic targets for DCR can be found in **Table 3**.

Potential Complications of Resuscitation

Abdominal trauma can affect specific organ systems, and the degree of trauma and required resuscitation can alter perfusion within the abdominal cavity. With fluid administration, the injured organs swell from the increased vascular volume. Any

Table 3
Therapeutic goals during damage control resuscitation[26]

	Without Neurotrauma	With Neurotrauma
Arterial pressure (mm Hg)	Before hemostasis: 80 ≤ systolic BP ≤ 100 After hemostasis: MAP ≥ 65	Before and after hemostasis: systolic BP ≥ 100 or MAP ≥ 80
Hemoglobin (g/dL)	7–9	7–9
INR	≤ 2	≤ 1.5
Platelet count/mm³	≥ 50,000	≥ 100,000
Calcium (mmol/dL)	≥ 10	
Fibrinogen (mg/dL)	150–200	
pH	> 7.2	
Temperature (°C)	≥ 36	

Abbreviations: BP, blood pressure; MAP, mean arterial blood pressure.

hemorrhage in the abdomen will contribute to the increasing cavity pressure. As the abdominal cavity pressure increases, the perfusion pressure to abdominal organs is compromised.

Bladder pressure has become the standard method of measuring intra-abdominal pressure (IAP). A foley catheter is placed in the bladder with the measurement transducer placed at the midaxillary line at the level of the iliac crest (**Fig. 5**).[27] A saline bolus, typically 25 to 50 mL depending on institutional-based protocols, is instilled through the foley and a pressure monitor is connected directly into the closed system. To ensure consistent pressure measurements, it is important to use the same amount of instilled volume every time the IAP is checked. Using different volumes may result in inconsistent readings between measurements.[28] IAP is measured during end-expiration in a supine and relaxed patient.[7] An IAP 5 to 7 mm Hg is typically considered normal in critically ill patients and less than 12 mm Hg is average. Intra-abdominal hypertension (IAH) is graded I to IV. Abdominal compartment syndrome (ACS) is defined as IAP greater than 20 mm Hg with associated organ dysfunction (**Table 4**).

ACS can be classified as primary, secondary, and recurrent. Primary ACS occurs from direct peritoneal or retroperitoneal injury or disease, and secondary ACS is caused by factors outside of the abdominal space.[29] Recurrent ACS is the re-

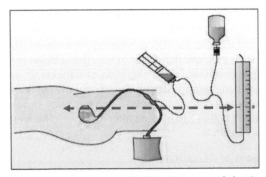

Fig. 5. Measuring bladder pressure. (Asencio C, Fleiszig Z. Intra-abdominal hypertension and ACS in acute pancreatitis. IntechOpen. https://www.intechopen.com/chapters/47645. Published March 4, 2015. Accessed September 6, 2022.)

Table 4 Intra-abdominal pressure grades[28]	
Grade	**Criteria**
I	IAP = 12–15 mm Hg
II	IAP = 16–20 mm Hg
III	IAP = 21–25 mm Hg
IV	IAP = > 25 mm Hg
ACS	IAP > 20 mm Hg with associated organ dysfunction

development of IAH after initiation of treatment of the primary or secondary cause. ACS is characterized by hypotension, refractory metabolic acidosis, oliguria, elevated peak airway pressures, hypoxemia, elevated serum lactate, and hypercapnia. As the abdominal pressure rises, perfusion to organs like the kidneys and intestines decreases and signs of organ dysfunction and failure develop. Diaphragmatic excursion can be impaired causing atelectasis, hypoxemia, hypercapnia, and respiratory failure.[30] Risk factors associated with the development of ACS include abdominal trauma, abdominal surgery, high volume resuscitation, gastrointestinal obstruction, major burn injuries, hypothermia, acidosis, ascites and peritoneal dialysis, mechanical ventilation, obesity, and sepsis.[29]

Management of Abdominal Compartment Syndrome

- Reduction of abdominal pressure and abdominal decompression
- Adjusting sedation and analgesia
- Neuromuscular blockade if appropriate
- Positioning
- Avoiding excessive volume administration
- Limiting restrictive clothing or dressings[27]

Decompression is achieved by inserting a nasogastric tube and placing to suction, rectal decompression, bladder decompression, and maintaining nothing per mouth (NPO) status. A decompressive laparotomy is a salvage technique for refractory ACS, though there is no uniform indication for a decompressive laparotomy. Recent studies suggest that early decompression has a mortality benefit, but there is no recommended timing of when to initiate the procedure. Additionally, there is no survival benefit seen with prophylactic laparotomy.[31]

ORGAN-SPECIFIC TRAUMA CONSIDERATIONS
Stomach

Penetrating gastric injuries are more prevalent than blunt mechanisms, usually from stabbings, gunshot wounds, and impalement. The stomach is a dynamic and flexible structure, which reduces the risk of trauma compared with solid organ structures. The stomach is also partially protected by the rib cage, providing some level of protection from blunt trauma.[32] Significant stomach injury is associated with concomitant organ injuries in 80% of cases.[33] Acute compression on the gastric wall during a blunt abdominal injury can cause an overdistention or crushing of the gastric mucosa, leading to rupture and mucosal destruction. Perforation can occur from penetrating objects and broken bones.[32] Rapid diagnosis and grading of gastric injuries are imperative, usually hallmarked by abdominal pain, tenderness to palpation, nausea, bloody emesis, peritoneal symptoms, and hemo/pneumoperitoneum on imaging.

Complications can arise from missed injuries, resulting in gastric spillage into the abdomen, abscess and fistula formation, peritonitis, and sepsis.[32]

Management

- Serial clinical assessments
- Diagnostic imaging with x-ray, ultrasound, and CT
- Surgical repair and gastric decompression
  - Surgical interventions typically involve primary repair of the injury, but resections are performed for higher-grade injuries[34]

Spleen

Splenic injuries are one of the most common solid abdominal organs injured after a traumatic event, occurring in nearly one-third of all abdominal traumas (**Table 5**). Splenic injuries occur from both blunt and penetrating mechanisms. Complications include subcapsular hematoma, splenic rupture, intra-abdominal hemorrhage, and pseudoaneurysm rupture.[35] Routine laboratory testing, such as CBC and lactate, and hemodynamic evaluations can help monitor for signs of hemorrhage and the

Table 5
Spleen injury scoring[34]

AAST Grade	Imaging/Pathologic Criteria	Operative Criteria
I	• Subcapsular hematoma < 10% surface area • Parenchymal Laceration < 1 cm in depth • Capsular tear	• Subcapsular hematoma < 10% surface area • Parenchymal Laceration < 1 cm in depth • Capsular tear
II	• Subcapsular hematoma 10%–50% surface area; interaparenchymal hematoma < 5 cm • Parenchymal laceration 1-3 cm in depth	• Subcapsular hematoma 10%–50% surface area; interaparenchymal hematoma < 5 cm • Parenchymal laceration 1-3 cm in depth
III	• Subcapsular hematoma >50% surface area; ruptured subcapsular or intraparenchymal hematoma ≥5 cm • Parenchymal Laceration > 3 cm in depth	• Subcapsular hematoma >50% surface area or expanding; ruptured subcapsular or intraparenchymal hematoma ≥5 cm • Parenchymal Laceration > 3 cm in depth
IV	• Any injury in the presence of a splenic vascular injury or active bleeding confined within splenic capsule • Parenchymal laceration involving segmental or hilar vessels producing >25% devascularization	• Parenchymal laceration involving segmental or hilar vessels producing >25% devascularization
V	• Any injury in the presence of splenic vascular injury with active bleeding extending beyond the spleen into the peritoneum • Shattered spleen	• Hilar vascular injury which devascularizes the spleen • Shattered spleen

Kozar, Rosemary A. MD, PhD; Crandall, Marie MD; Shanmuganathan, Kathirkamanthan MD; Zarzaur, Ben L. MD; Coburn, Mike MD; Cribari, Chris MD; Kaups, Krista MD; Schuster, Kevin MD; Tominaga, Gail T. MD; the AAST Patient Assessment Committee. Organ injury scaling 2018 update: Spleen, liver, and kidney. Journal of Trauma and Acute Care Surgery 85(6):p 1119-1122, December 2018. | DOI: 10.1097/TA.0000000000002058.

need for surgical intervention. CT of the spleen is considered the gold standard for diagnostic imaging. Ultrasound evaluation can also help classify the degree of injury and prompt type of management (eg, nonoperative management, angiogram, and angioembolization, or surgical intervention).[36]

Management

- Nonoperative management on hemodynamically stable patients who lack peritoneal symptoms and are able to be closely monitored
- The medical facility should have an available operating room if an urgent laparotomy is required
- Nonoperative management requires frequent assessments in a highly monitored setting and includes serial abdominal examinations, laboratories, and bedrest
- Patients are at high risk of clinical decompensation if their CT has a vascular blush, pseudoaneurysm, grade III injuries with large hemoperitoneum, or a grade IV or V injury[37]

Pancreas

Pancreatic trauma occurs in less than 1% of all trauma cases, but can be seen in up to 11% of all abdominal trauma.[38] The Pancreas Injury Scale grades injuries from I to V. Grade I is a hematoma with a minor contusion or laceration without ductal injury. Grade II reflects a major hematoma or laceration without ductal injury. Grade III is described as a distal transection or parenchymal injury involving the duct. Grade IV is a proximal transection of injury involving the ampulla. Lastly, grade V reflects complete disruption of the pancreatic head.[38]

Complications from pancreatic injuries include pancreatic leak, abscess and fistula formation, pancreatitis, and acute hemorrhage. A CT scan is the primary method of imaging pancreatic injury, with magnetic resonance cholangiopancreatography and endoscopic retrograde cholangiopancreatography being alternative options for evaluation.[39]

Genitourinary Trauma

Genitourinary (GU) trauma can be seen in blunt and PAT and is found in 10% to 18% of all abdominal trauma cases. Direct kidney injury is present in nearly 25% of all abdominal trauma.[40] Evaluating injury to the kidneys, ureters, bladder, and urethra involves clinical monitoring of urine production and quality, signs of obstruction and hemorrhage, laboratory testing, and radiology imaging. Renal injuries are graded according to the American Associated for the Surgery of Trauma (AAST) classification and can vary between grades I and V (**Table 6**).[34] Bladder trauma is typically caused by rupture after a compressive injury (ie, seatbelt injury during a motor vehicle crash) or perforation (from bullet wounds and pelvic bone fractures).[40]

Clinical assessment after GU trauma should include pelvic or pubic tenderness, ecchymosis, penetrating injuries, distention, subjective urgency, dysuria, or hematuria.[7] FAST examination can evaluate for renal contusion and hemoperitoneum.[2] Clinical symptoms may rule in or rule out certain conditions. Unilateral flank or costovertebral tenderness may accompany injuries to the renal structure.[7] Symptoms of inability to void, urinary urgency, dysuria, or spasmodic pain with incontinence can all be signs of lower urinary tract injuries. Urinary analysis can detect the presence of red blood cells and protein in the urine caused by renal laceration or contusion, bladder rupture, and damage to the ureters or urethra.[7] Imaging of the GU tract includes a CT scan with intravenous (IV) contrast, and delayed phase contrast-imaging can evaluate ureteral injury by detecting extravasation into the abdominal cavity.[40] Cystograms and cystoscopies can evaluate the bladder structure and

Table 6
Kidney injury scoring[34]

AAST Grade	Imaging/Pathologic Criteria	Operative Criteria
I	• Subcapsular hematoma or parenchymal contusion without parenchymal laceration	• Nonexpanding subcapsular hematoma • Parenchymal contusion without laceration
II	• Perirenal hematoma confined to Gerota fascia • Renal parenchymal laceration ≤ 1 cm depth without urinary extravasation	• Nonexpanding perirenal hematoma confined to Gerota fascia • Renal parenchymal laceration ≤ 1 cm depth without urinary extravasation
III	• Renal parenchymal laceration>1 cm depth without collecting system rupture or urinary extravasation • Any injury in the presence of a kidney vascular injury or active bleeding contained within Gerota fascia	• Renal parenchymal laceration>1 cm depth without collecting system rupture or urinary extravasation
IV	• Parenchymal laceration extending into urinary collecting system with urinary extravasation • Renal pelvis laceration and/or complete ureteropelvic disruption • Segmental renal vein or artery injury • Active bleeding beyond Gerota fascia into the retroperitoneum or peritoneum • Segmental or complete kidney infarction(s) due to vessel thrombosis without active bleeding	• Parenchymal laceration extending into urinary collecting system with urinary extravasation • Renal pelvis laceration and/or complete ureteropelvic disruption • Segmental renal vein or artery injury • Segmental or complete kidney infarction(s) due to vessel thrombosis without active bleeding
V	• Main renal artery or vein laceration or avulsion of hilum • Devascularized kidney with active bleeding • Shattered kidney with loss of identifiable parenchymal renal anatomy	• Main renal artery or vein laceration or avulsion of hilum • Devascularized kidney • Shattered kidney with loss of identifiable parenchymal renal anatomy

Kozar, Rosemary A. MD, PhD; Crandall, Marie MD; Shanmuganathan, Kathirkamanthan MD; Zarzaur, Ben L. MD; Coburn, Mike MD; Cribari, Chris MD; Kaups, Krista MD; Schuster, Kevin MD; Tominaga, Gail T. MD; the AAST Patient Assessment Committee. Organ injury scaling 2018 update: Spleen, liver, and kidney. Journal of Trauma and Acute Care Surgery 85(6):p 1119-1122, December 2018. | DOI: 10.1097/TA.0000000000002058.

ureteral pathways. High-grade GU injuries should prompt the surgical team to evaluate for other organ damage, as isolated GU injuries rarely occur.[41]

Any clinical symptom of active hemorrhage, hemodynamic instability, or progressive abdominal distention should prompt an urgent surgical evaluation for hemorrhage control, primary repair, nephrectomy, or urinary diversion. Many GU injuries are managed nonoperatively, as recent data suggest there is a mortality benefit in avoiding unnecessary laparotomies and nephrectomies.[42]

Table 7 Duodenal injury scale[34]		
AAST Grade	**Injury Type**	**Injury Description**
I	• Hematoma • Laceration	• Involves a single portion of duodenum • Partial thickness injury to duodenum without perforation
II	• Hematoma • Laceration	• Involves more than a single portion of duodenum • Disruption to < 50% of lumen circumference
III	• Laceration	• Disruption 50%–75% of circumference to D2 • Disruption 50%–100% of circumference to D2, D3, or D4
IV	• Laceration	• Disruption > 75% of circumference of D2 • Involves ampulla or distal common bile duct
V	• Laceration • Vascular	• Massive destruction of duodenopancreatic structures • Devascularized duodenum

Adapted from Moore, Ernest E. MD; Jurkovich, Gregory J. MD; Knudson, M. Margaret MD; Cogbill, Thomas H. MD; Malangoni, Mark A. MD; Champion, Howard R. MD; Shackford, Steven R. MD. Organ Injury Scaling VI: Extrahepatic Biliary, Esophagus, Stomach, Vulva, Vagina, Uterus (Nonpregnant), Uterus (Pregnant), Fallopian Tube, and Ovary. The Journal of Trauma: Injury, Infection, and Critical Care 39(6):p 1069-1070, December 1995.

Small and Large Bowel

Adult duodenal injuries (**Table 7**) account for nearly 5% of all abdominal traumatic injuries and hollow viscus and mesenteric injuries are seen in up to 17% of cases.[43] Major vascular damage is associated with 23% to 40% of patients with intestinal trauma. CT is the preferred imaging technique to evaluate for bowel injury. Intravenous contrast may be considered when evaluating vascular structures and perforations, and is usually sufficient to evaluate the bowel after BAT. Oral contrast may be considered when investigating luminal obstructions and perforations. Rectal contrast is also considered when evaluating descending colonic and rectal injuries.[43] Clinicians should also be aware that CT scans have a false-negative rate of up to 20% for bowel injury, and clinical monitoring should be followed despite a negative CT reading.[43,44]

The use of the FAST examination and DPL may offer clues to the presence of bowel injury, with positive results prompting surgical intervention. Negative results for the FAST and DPL examinations do not specifically rule out injury and serial abdominal examinations should be conducted for at least 24 hours.[44] Any radiologic evidence of extraluminal air, enteral contrast leak, or bowel wall defects should prompt a surgical evaluation.[43,45]

Hemodynamic stability is the key factor when determining nonoperative versus surgical intervention for blunt abdominal injuries. Management of bowel injuries can usually be conservative with serial abdominal examinations in blunt duodenal injuries with grade I or II injuries that are hemodynamically stable.[44] Hallmark signs and symptoms of progressive bowel injury include

- Abdominal pain
- Tenderness to palpation
- Abdominal distention
- Nausea or emesis
- Hypotension
- Worsening lactatemia
- Ongoing leukocytosis

Table 8
Colon injury scale[34]

AAST Grade	Injury Type	Injury Description
I	• Hematoma • Laceration	• Contusion or hematoma without devascularization • Partial thickness injury without perforation
II	• Hematoma • Laceration	• Laceration <50% of colonic circumference
III	• Laceration	• Laceration > or equal to 50% of colonic circumference, without transaction
IV	• Laceration	• Transection of the colon
V	• Laceration • Vascular	• Transection of the colon with segmental tissue loss • Devascularized colonic segment

Adapted from Moore, Ernest E. MD; Jurkovich, Gregory J. MD; Knudson, M. Margaret MD; Cogbill, Thomas H. MD; Malangoni, Mark A. MD; Champion, Howard R. MD; Shackford, Steven R. MD. Organ Injury Scaling VI: Extrahepatic Biliary, Esophagus, Stomach, Vulva, Vagina, Uterus (Nonpregnant), Uterus (Pregnant), Fallopian Tube, and Ovary. The Journal of Trauma: Injury, Infection, and Critical Care 39(6):p 1069-1070, December 1995.

Any perforating injury, hemodynamic instability, or peritoneal symptoms should prompt a surgical evaluation.[38] If there is identified bowel injury, further evaluation should be performed to investigate injury to the liver, biliary tree, pancreas, stomach, and colon (**Table 8**). Patients with altered levels of consciousness, spinal cord injury, or requiring sedation should be considered for surgical evaluation regardless of hemodynamic stability. In PAT, surgical exploration is typically indicated for a full evaluation of intestinal injuries in unstable patients.[46] Surgical control may involve a damage control approach and surgical repair can involve a primary repair, resection of injured bowel with anastomosis, diversion to an ostomy, and a delayed definitive reconstruction.[44,45,47]

Liver

The liver is commonly injured in blunt and PAT and can cause major concerns due to the highly vascular parenchyma.[7] Liver injuries are graded according to the AAST Liver Injury Scoring scale (**Table 9**).[48] Nonoperative management has become the standard of care for minor- and moderate-grade injuries (I–III), and high-grade injuries (IV–V) can also be managed nonoperatively if the patient is hemodynamically stable. The initial clinical examination should include the primary trauma survey and evaluation of symptoms (right upper quadrant pain, tenderness, ecchymosis, penetrating wounds, distention), and hemodynamic monitoring. An abdominal FAST examination can be performed to assess for hemoperitoneum, but a CT scan with IV contrast is considered the gold standard for evaluating hepatic injuries.[49]

Hemodynamic instability usually warrants a surgical evaluation, and nonoperative management should only be considered in areas where immediate access to an operating room is available if clinical deterioration occurs. Angiography and angioembolization are common methods of controlling hepatic hemorrhage in patients who have contrast extravasation on their CT imaging. Surgical interventions may include primary repair, DCS and wound packing, and hepatic lobe resection. In extremely severe cases, complete hepatectomy may be required due to organ injury but a liver transplant would also be required.[49]

Table 9 Liver scoring table[34]		
AAST Grade	**Imaging/Pathologic Criteria**	**Operative Criteria**
I	• Subcapsular hematoma < 10% surface area • Parenchymal laceration < 1 cm in depth	• Subcapsular hematoma < 10% surface area • Parenchymal laceration < 1 cm in depth • Capsular tear
II	• Subcapsular hematoma 10%–50% surface area; intraparenchymal hematoma < 10 cm in diameter • Parenchymal laceration 1-3 cm in depth and ≤ 10 cm length	• Subcapsular hematoma 10%–50% surface area; intraparenchymal hematoma < 10 cm in diameter • Parenchymal laceration 1-3 cm in depth and ≤ 10 cm length
III	• Subcapsular hematoma >50% surface area; ruptured subcapsular or parenchymal hematoma • Intraparenchymal hematoma > 10 cm • Laceration > 3 cm depth • Any injury in the presence of a liver vascular injury or active bleeding contained within liver parenchyma	• Subcapsular hematoma >50% surface area or expanding ruptured subcapsular or parenchymal hematoma • Intraparenchymal hematoma > 10 cm • Laceration > 3 cm depth
IV	• Parenchymal disruption involving 25%–75% of a hepatic lobe • Active bleeding extending beyond the liver parenchyma into the peritoneum	• Parenchymal disruption involving 25%–75% of a hepatic lobe
V	• Parenchymal disruption > 75% of hepatic lobe • Juxtahepatic venous injury to include retrohepatic vena cava and central major hepatic veins	• Parenchymal disruption > 75% of hepatic lobe • Juxtahepatic venous injury to include retrohepatic vena cava and central major hepatic veins

Kozar, Rosemary A. MD, PhD; Crandall, Marie MD; Shanmuganathan, Kathirkamanthan MD; Zarzaur, Ben L. MD; Coburn, Mike MD; Cribari, Chris MD; Kaups, Krista MD; Schuster, Kevin MD; Tominaga, Gail T. MD; the AAST Patient Assessment Committee. Organ injury scaling 2018 update: Spleen, liver, and kidney. Journal of Trauma and Acute Care Surgery 85(6):p 1119-1122, December 2018. | DOI: 10.1097/TA.0000000000002058.

Management

- Serial clinical examinations aimed at monitoring for ongoing hemorrhage and the development of ACS
- Hemodynamic monitoring
- Laboratory assessments of hepatic function, complete blood count, lactate, and coagulation panel
- Monitoring for ongoing hemorrhage and biliary leakage and output from surgical drain sites drains
- Major liver injuries should also prompt the trauma team to adjust medication types and dosages to avoid hepatotoxic agents

Vascular Trauma

Vascular trauma is the leading cause of death from trauma and in-hospital mortality rates range from 12% to 28%.[50] Most injuries are to arterial vessels and are usually concomitant with other organ injuries. DCR should be initiated in all hemodynamically unstable patients and the primary objective for the medical team should be prompt identification of hemorrhagic injuries. The ATLS protocol is the standard of care when managing traumatic vascular injuries.[7] Courses such as the American College of Surgeons' STOP THE BLEED are widely available and train nonmedical bystanders and medical professionals to control hemorrhage.[51]

Evaluation of vascular trauma includes a clinical assessment of hemorrhage, manual palpation of pulses, and monitoring for signs of ischemia. Any visible and life-threatening bleeding should have pressure immediately applied; the use of a tourniquet and wound packing can help stabilize bleeding until definitive management is implemented. Vascular injury should be assumed in any hemodynamically unstable patient until ruled out, and operative management is the standard of care for all unstable vascular trauma. Ultrasound imaging can quickly evaluate for vascular and organ hemorrhage, and computed tomography angiography is recommended to evaluate for bleeding in hemodynamically stable patients. Obtaining a medical history and medication list is important for the consideration of bleeding disorders and anticoagulant medication reversal.[50] The initial presence of hemodynamic stability should not rule out the presence of major bleeding, as 30% of patients present as stable but then progress to hemorrhagic shock.[50] The serial use of FAST examinations, neurovascular assessments, hemodynamic monitoring, and laboratory testing should be routinely used to monitor clinical stability and hemorrhage control.

Unstable patients may require exploratory surgery before formal imaging being obtained. Techniques used to manage vascular injuries include primary repair, angioplasty and grafting, vascular ligation, and angioembolization. Supportive care and targeted resuscitation should be guided by DCR principles and massive transfusion protocols can be used to quickly obtain blood products for transfusion. Resuscitative endovascular balloon occlusion of the aorta is an occlusive technique used to stop bleeding by temporarily inflating a vascular balloon within zones of the aorta to target specific sites of arterial bleeding until definitive surgical management can be accomplished.[50]

SUMMARY

Abdominal trauma is associated with significant morbidity and mortality rates and understanding the mechanism can help guide the care team during their assessment and development of a plan. On arrival at the hospital, the care team should follow the ATLS primary survey principles and prompt surgical exploration should occur if the patient is hemodynamically unstable or has clinical evidence of massive hemorrhage. Permissive hypotension, fluid restriction, and balanced transfusion strategy concepts of DCR should be followed during the resuscitative phase. The utilization of various imaging techniques, physical examination, and hemodynamic monitoring allows for prompt diagnosis and surgical control. Collaboration and effective communication are essential in the management of these critically injured patients.

CLINICS CARE POINTS

- Prompt reversal and prevention of hypothermia, coagulopathy, and acidosis
- Follow the concepts of DCR: fluid restriction, balanced transfusion strategy, and reverse coagulopathy
- Maintaining hemodynamic stability (target normal BP parameters once hemostasis has been achieved)

- Assessment of laboratory values including H/H, coagulation studies, and TEG or ROTEM
- Thorough and repeated physical examinations should be performed to monitor for clinical deterioration

DISCLOSURE

There are no conflicts of interest or financial gains to disclose for either author.

REFERENCES

1. World Health Organization. Injuries and violence. World Health Organization; 2021. Available at: www.who.int/news-room/fact-sheets/detail/injuries-and-violence. Accessed 20 Aug. 2022.
2. Boutros SM, Nassef MA, Abdel-Ghany AF. Blunt abdominal trauma: the role of focused abdominal sonography in assessment of organ injury and reducing the need for CT. Alexandria J. Med 2016;52(1):35–41.
3. Akeel AS, Mahdi BA, Alshammasi ZA, et al. Emergency assessment and management of abdominal trauma. 2021. Available at: https://www.ecronicon.com/ecmi/pdf/ECMI-17-01041.pdf. Accessed May 15, 2022.
4. Hanna K, Asmar S, Ditillo M, et al. Readmission with major abdominal complications after penetrating abdominal trauma. J Surg Res 2021;257:69–78.
5. Durso AM, Paes FM, Caban K, et al. Evaluation of penetrating abdominal and pelvic trauma. Eur J Radiol 2020;130:109187.
6. Solanki Hardik J, Patel Himanshu R. Blunt abdomen trauma: a study of 50 cases. Int Surg 2018;5:1763–9.
7. American College of Surgeons. Advanced trauma life support (ATLS®): the tenth edition. J Trauma and Acute Care Surgery 2018;82–100.
8. Lotfollahzadeh S, Burns B. Penetrating abdominal trauma. StatPearls. Available at: https://www.ncbi.nlm.nih.gov/books/NBK459123/. Published June 3, 2022. Accessed September 6, 2022.
9. Arumugam S, Al-Hassani A, El-Menyar A, et al. Frequency, causes and pattern of abdominal trauma: a 4-year descriptive analysis. J Emerg Trauma Shock 2015; 8(4):193–8.
10. Forbes J, Burns B. Abdominal gunshot wounds. StatPearls. Available at: https://www.ncbi.nlm.nih.gov/books/NBK564335/. Accessed September 6, 2022.
11. Boukerrouche A. Damage control surgery concept. J Trauma 2019;3(1):6–9.
12. Kornblith AE, Addo N, Plasencia M, et al. Development of a consensus-based definition of focused assessment with sonography for trauma in children. JAMA Netw Open 2022;5(3):e222922. Published 2022 Mar 1.
13. Schellenberg M, Owattanapanich N, Emigh B, et al. Contemporary utility of diagnostic peritoneal aspiration in trauma. J Trauma Acute Care Surg 2021;91(5):814–9.
14. Hooper N, Armstrong T. Hemorrhagic shock. StatPearls. Available at: https://www.ncbi.nlm.nih.gov/books/NBK470382/. Published July 11, 2022. Accessed September 6, 2022.
15. Garcia A. Critical care issues in the early management of severe trauma. Surg Clin North Am 2006;86(6):1359–87.
16. Kelley KC, Dammann K, Alers A, et al. Resuscitation endpoints in traumatic shock: a focused review with emphasis on point-of-care approaches [Online first]. IntechOpen 2020. https://doi.org/10.5772/intechopen.90686.

17. Shagana JA, Dhanraj M, Jain AR, et al. (PDF) hypovolemic shock - a review. ResearchGate. Available at: https://www.researchgate.net/publication/328567156_Hypovolemic_shock_-_A_review. Published July 2018. Accessed September 6, 2022.

18. Dutton RP. Resuscitative strategies to maintain homeostasis during damage control surgery. Br J Surg 2012;99(Suppl 1):21–8.

19. Leibner E, Andreae M, Galvagno SM, et al. Damage control resuscitation. Clin Exp Emerg Med 2020;7(1):5–13.

20. Spahn DR, Bouillon B, Cerny V, et al. The European guideline on management of major bleeding and coagulopathy following trauma: fifth edition. Crit Care 2019; 23(1). https://doi.org/10.1186/s13054-019-2347-3.

21. Giannoudi M, Harwood P. Damage control resuscitation: lessons learned. Eur J Trauma Emerg Surg 2016;42:273–82.

22. Cantle PM, Roberts DJ, Holcomb JB. Damage control resuscitation across the phases of major injury care. Curr Trauma Rep 2017;3(3):238–48.

23. Heim C, Steurer M, Brohi K. Damage control resuscitation: more than just transfusion strategies. Curr Anesthesiol Rep 2016;6(1):72–8.

24. Rotondo MF, Schwab CW, McGonigal MD, et al. Damage control': an approach for improved survival in exsanguinating penetrating abdominal injury. J Trauma 1993;35(3):375–83.

25. Roberts I, Shakur H, Coats T, et al. The crash-2 trial: a randomised controlled trial and economic evaluation of the effects of tranexamic acid on death, Vascular occlusive events and transfusion requirement in bleeding trauma patients. Health Technol Assess 2013;17(10). https://doi.org/10.3310/hta17100.

26. Malgras B, Prunet B, Lesaffre X, et al. Damage control: concept and implementation. J Visc Surg 2017;154(Suppl 1):S19-S29.

27. Asencio C, Fleiszig Z. Intra-abdominal hypertension and abdominal compartment syndrome in acute pancreatitis. IntechOpen. Available at: https://www.intechopen.com/chapters/47645. Published March 4, 2015. Accessed September 6, 2022.

28. Kirkpatrick A, De Waele J, Roberts D, et al. WSACS consensus guidelines summary. World society of the abdominal compartment syndrome. Available at: http://www.wsacs.org/education/436/wsacs-consensus-guidelines-summary/. Published April 7, 2021. Accessed September 6, 2022.

29. Gray S, Christensen M, Craft J. The gastro-renal effects of intra-abdominal hypertension: implications for critical care nurses. Intensive Crit Care Nurs 2018;48: 69–74.

30. Vatankhah S, Sheikhi RA, Heidari M, et al. The relationship between fluid resuscitation and intra-abdominal hypertension in patients with blunt abdominal trauma. Int J Crit Illn Inj Sci 2018;8(3):149–53.

31. Kirkpatrick AW, Roberts DJ, De Waele J, et al. Intra-abdominal hypertension and the abdominal compartment syndrome: updated consensus definitions and clinical practice guidelines from the World Society of the Abdominal Compartment Syndrome. Intensive Care Med 2013;39(7):1190–206.

32. Aboobakar MR, Singh JP, Maharaj K, et al. Gastric perforation following blunt abdominal trauma. Trauma Case Rep 2017;10:12–5.

33. Allen N, Kong V, Cheung C, et al. Laparotomy for penetrating gastric trauma - a South African experience. Injury 2022;53(5):1610–4.

34. Moore E, et al, Malangoni M, et al. Injury scoring scale. The American association for the surgery of trauma. Available at: https://www.aast.org/resources-detail/injury-scoring-scale. Published May 4, 2021. Accessed September 6, 2022.

35. Lee JT, Slade E, Uyeda J, et al. American society of emergency radiology multi-center blunt splenic trauma study: CT and clinical findings. Radiology 2021; 299(1):122–30.
36. Coccolini F, Montori G, Catena F, et al. Splenic trauma: WSES classification and guidelines for adult and pediatric patients. World J Emerg Surg 2017;12:40.
37. Stassen NA, Bhullar I, Cheng JD, et al. Selective nonoperative management of blunt splenic injury: an Eastern Association for the Surgery of Trauma practice management guideline. J Trauma Acute Care Surg 2012;73(5 Suppl 4): S294–300.
38. Coccolini F, Kobayashi L, Kluger Y, et al. Duodeno-pancreatic and extrahepatic biliary tree trauma: WSES-AAST guidelines. World J Emerg Surg 2019;14(1). https://doi.org/10.1186/s13017-019-0278-6.
39. Ho VP, Patel NJ, Bokhari F, et al. Management of adult pancreatic injuries: a practice management guideline from the Eastern Association for the Surgery of Trauma. J Trauma Acute Care Surg 2017;82(1):185–99.
40. Leite C, Guerreiro N, Camerin GR, et al. A practical guide to genitourinary trauma. Radiographics 2021;41(1):96–7.
41. Coccolini F, Moore EE, Kluger Y, et al. Kidney and uro-trauma: WSES-AAST guidelines. World J Emerg Surg 2019;14:54.
42. West A, Gan C. Genitourinary trauma. Surgery 2022;40(8):540–9.
43. Smyth L, Bendinelli C, Lee N, et al. WSES guidelines on blunt and penetrating bowel injury: diagnosis, investigations, and treatment. World J Emerg Surg 2022;17(1):13. Published 2022 Mar 4.
44. McMahon K, Balasubramanya R. Intestinal trauma. StatPearls. Available at: https://www.ncbi.nlm.nih.gov/books/NBK557624/. Published 2022. Accessed September 6, 2022.
45. Weinberg JA, Peck KA, Ley EJ, et al. Evaluation and management of bowel and mesenteric injuries after blunt trauma: a Western Trauma Association critical decisions algorithm. J Trauma Acute Care Surg 2021;91(5):903–8.
46. Como JJ, Bokhari F, Chiu WC, et al. Practice management guidelines for selective nonoperative management of penetrating abdominal trauma. J Trauma 2010; 68(3):721–33.
47. Biffl WL, Moore EE, Feliciano DV, et al. Management of colorectal injuries: a Western Trauma Association critical decisions algorithm. J Trauma Acute Care Surg 2018;85(5):1016–20.
48. Kozar RA, Crandall M, Shanmuganathan K, et al. Organ injury scaling 2018 update: spleen, liver, and kidney. J Trauma Acute Care Surg 2018;85(6):1119–22 [published correction appears in J Trauma Acute Care Surg;87(2):512].
49. Coccolini F, Coimbra R, Ordonez C, et al. Liver trauma: WSES 2020 guidelines. World J Emerg Surg 2020;15(1):24.
50. Kobayashi L, Coimbra R, Goes AMO Jr, et al. American Association for the Surgery of Trauma-World Society of Emergency Surgery guidelines on diagnosis and management of abdominal vascular injuries. J Trauma Acute Care Surg 2020; 89(6):1197–211.
51. American College of Surgeons. Stop the bleed. Stop the bleed. Available at: http://www.stopthebleed.org/. Accessed September 6, 2022.

Trauma in the Obstetric Patient

Halli Carr, DNP, APRN, ACNP-BC*, Renee' Jones, DNP, APRN, WHNP-BC

KEYWORDS

- Bleeding • Maternal–fetal • Obstetrics • Pregnancy • Trauma

KEY POINTS

- Trauma during pregnancy presents a unique challenge because there are two patients to consider during assessment and resuscitation.
- Assessment of the pregnant trauma patient should follow the same systematic guidelines as other trauma patients with a few additional considerations.
- Priority should be on maternal resuscitation as fetal outcomes depend on maternal well-being. The severity of maternal injuries determines maternal and fetal outcome.
- The early recognition of pregnancy complications and early involvement of specialists such as obstetrics and gynecology (OBGYN) or maternal fetal medicine (MFM) are the key to preventing maternal–fetal complications.
- Given the risk of isoimmunization with small amounts of blood transfer, all pregnant Rh-negative trauma patients should receive Rh immunoglobulin therapy unless the injury is remote from the uterus.

TRAUMA IN THE OBSTETRIC PATIENT

Trauma affects a significant population each year worldwide. Within the umbrella of trauma, there are several special populations to consider, one of them being the obstetric patient. Roughly, one in 12 pregnancies is affected by trauma.[1] In addition, trauma is the leading nonobstetric cause of maternal and fetal mortality/morbidity.[2] Common traumatic events affecting pregnant patients include motor vehicle collisions (MVCs), falls, assaults/intimate partner violence (IPV), and suicide. A recent systematic review found that IPV, including verbal violence, is reported to occur in up to 57% of all pregnancies.[3] When the pregnant trauma victim presents to the emergency department, it is important that the care provided is multidisciplinary in scope. This article discuss trauma during pregnancy and the manifestations unique to the pregnant trauma victim.

The authors have no significant financial or professional disclosures.
Baylor Louise Herrington School of Nursing, 333 North Washington Avenue, Dallas, TX 75246, USA
* Corresponding author.
E-mail address: Halli_carr@baylor.edu

Crit Care Nurs Clin N Am 35 (2023) 213–222
https://doi.org/10.1016/j.cnc.2023.02.012
0899-5885/23/© 2023 Elsevier Inc. All rights reserved.

INTRODUCTION

Care of the pregnant patient with traumatic injuries requires special knowledge and understanding. Obstetric patients represent a vulnerable population demanding increased consideration and focus in their care due to the changes in anatomy and physiology that occur as a result of pregnancy. These patients are at risk for all common traumatic injuries as well as pregnancy-specific injuries such as placental abruption, uterine rupture, and preterm labor. Dalton and colleagues also found that maternal trauma in the first trimester is associated with a significantly increased risk of placental dysfunction later in pregnancy.[4] Thus, even if there are no immediate complications from the traumatic event itself, pregnant patients who experience trauma early in the pregnancy will require antenatal surveillance for late complications down the road. Finally, obstetric patients also present a greater emotional challenge to the care team as two patients are represented, rather than just one.

MATERNAL PHYSIOLOGIC ADAPTATIONS RELATED TO TRAUMA

Depending on gestational age, the anatomic and physiologic changes in pregnancy may affect the patient's response to traumatic injury. The changes in pregnancy may mask the ability of the health care provider to accurately diagnose traumatic injuries and provide appropriate treatment. The most important physiologic changes in pregnancy as it relates to trauma will be discussed.

Cardiovascular Alterations

One of the most dynamic physiologic changes influencing pregnancy and trauma outcomes is the increase in blood and plasma volume. The cardiovascular system is at a high-output, low-resistance state. This process starts as the red cell volume increases by 30% and the plasma volume increases by 50%, thereby creating a hemodilutional anemia effect by late term.[5] The changes take effect by the end of the first trimester and peak by 28 to 32 weeks of gestation.[5] Cardiac output increases due to the increase in heart rate and stroke volume. At term, the normal cardiac output in pregnancy is 6 to 7 L per minute.[6] The resting heart rate increases 15 to 20 beats per minute over nonpregnant values. These changes assist in increasing the blood flow to the uterus and growing fetus. Every 8 to 11 minutes, the entire maternal blood system has circulated through the uteroplacental system; thus, hemorrhage in the pregnant trauma patient can result in significant fetal compromise and even death.[5]

Owing to the effect of increased progesterone levels, systemic vascular resistance and blood pressure are decreased. This directly results from vasodilation of the peripheral vessels along with a low-resistance placental vascular system. It is essential to maintain an adequate arterial blood pressure to preserve uterine blood flow. The peak time that these hemodynamic changes take effect is during the second trimester, and as a result, the placenta receives the majority of the cardiac output at this time. By the end of the third trimester, the maternal blood pressure levels return to the prepregnancy state.

Owing to the hypervolemic state of pregnancy, the trauma team must keep in mind that the pregnant woman may not show signs of hypovolemia or hemodynamic compromise until she has lost at least 30% to 40% of her blood volume.[7] Once the patient demonstrates tachycardia and low blood pressure, the team is already behind in volume resuscitation and the fetus is likely in distress. If there is a significant amount of fluid loss, the uterus is a nonessential organ and blood flow will be shunted. If this occurs, the fetus will be without blood and oxygen. Frequently in late pregnancy, the first hemodynamic sign of volume loss is manifested by fetal distress.

Positioning of the pregnant trauma patient can directly affect the cardiac output. The best position for the pregnant patient is the lateral position. When providing care to the pregnant trauma patient, it is best to tilt the pregnant patient using a hip wedge if the patient should need to be supine. While lying supine, the gravid uterus compresses the inferior vena cava (IVC) causing decreased cardiac output and decreased uteroplacental perfusion. This can exacerbate hypotension and shock states and foil resuscitation.

Pulmonary and Respiratory Changes

As the uterus rises, the diaphragm elevates by 4 cm causing the length of the lungs to decrease.[5] Thus, the residual capacity of the lungs is diminished. In addition, the anterior posterior diameter of the chest increases. Should a chest tube need to be placed for a pregnant trauma patient, the insertion point should be the third or fourth intercostal space to avoid injuring the diaphragm.

The pregnant patient increases their minute ventilation at least 40% by term due to the increased respiratory rate and expanding tidal volume, thereby decreasing the arterial carbon dioxide concentration.[5] These changes cause the pregnant woman to have a decreased oxygen reserve, decreased blood-buffering capacity, increased oxygen consumption, and decreased functional residual capacity which results in a state of compensated respiratory alkalemia. This sets the stage for the pregnant woman to quickly become hypoxic and unable to compensate when for associated acidemia. Should the patient need to be ventilated, it is important to maintain this compensated respiratory alkalosis as transfer of oxygen and carbon dioxide occurs to the fetus under these conditions.

Hematological Changes

As a result of the greater increase in plasma volume compared with red blood cell volume, a hemodilutional anemia occurs. This produces lower hematocrit and hemoglobin values for pregnant patients. The normal range for a hematocrit in an obstetric patient is 31.9% to 36.5%.[5] In addition, the pregnant woman exists in a prothrombotic state and holds onto clot longer. This hypercoagulable state occurs due to increases in factors VII, VIII, IX, X, and fibrinogen. The pregnant woman also has a decreased ability for fibrinolysis or clot breakdown. These natural-occurring changes in clotting exist as a physiologic mechanism to prevent hemorrhage with birth. Trauma is also a prothrombotic state; therefore, pregnant trauma patients are at increased risk for clotting events and disseminated intravascular coagulation (DIC). Finally, during pregnancy, the white blood cell count is generally 10,000/μL and can increase to as high as 25,000/μL in response to stress or labor.[5]

Gastrointestinal Changes

The small bowel is displaced into the upper abdomen as a result of the enlarging uterus. Other organs in the abdomen maybe displaced cephalad as well, so it is important to recognize potential altered patterns of injury in the pregnant trauma patient. Furthermore, due to the progesterone causing relaxation of the smooth muscle, gastric emptying is delayed. This increases the potential for reflux and aspiration of stomach contents into the lungs. Therefore, it is important to consider early placement of a nasogastric tube for gastric decompression and use of other maneuvers such as cricoid pressure during airway attempts.

Genitourinary Changes

The ureters and renal pelvis are dilated due to relaxation of the smooth muscle from progesterone as well as compression from the uterus. This may create a physiologic hydronephrosis of pregnancy. Owing to the dilated ureters, dilated renal pelvis, and compression from the gravid uterus, stasis of urine is common. These changes lead to an increased frequency of bacteremia or pyelonephritis in the pregnant patient. In addition, the glomerular filtration rate (GFR) is increased causing an increase in creatinine level, urea, and uric acid. A normal serum creatinine as found in a nonpregnant patient would be consistent with compromised renal function in the pregnant patient. During pregnancy, urine output is increased, yet urine-specific gravity is decreased. Serum protein decreases due to the increase in GFR. Last, the bladder is susceptible to injury due to displacement during pregnancy as it is moved upward and forward out of the protection of the pelvis.

Uterus

At 12 weeks, the uterus rises above the symphysis pubis and into the abdomen, which makes it vulnerable to injury from blunt or penetrating abdominal trauma. Owing to the uterus' presence in the abdomen, it is more directly susceptible to abruptio placenta from blunt impact such as from motor vehicle collisions, falls, or IPV. One must consider also that the uterus is more likely to hemorrhage during abdominal trauma due to the increased blood flow increasing risk of hypovolemia in pregnant trauma patients.

APPROACH
Assessment of the Pregnant Trauma Patient

Primary survey (ABCDE)
Advanced trauma life support and trauma nursing-specific certifications (trauma certified registered nurse [TCRN], trauma nursing core course [TNCC]) emphasize a systematic, organized approach to the primary survey using the ABCDE algorithm.[8]

- A: Airway maintenance and cervical spine protection

Examine the airway while maintaining cervical spine immobilization. Use jaw thrust maneuvers as needed to visualize the oral airway. Airways can be difficult in pregnancy due to the increase in progesterone. They can also have easier bleeding in the airways as a result of this. Always have advanced airway maneuvers available (GlideScope, smaller-sized endotracheal tubes, surgical airway equipment) and have the most experienced provider attempt airway placement.

- B: Breathing and ventilation

If at all possible, maintain the patient in an upright position to displace the uterus distally and allow the diaphragm to fully expand. If there is concern for spinal injury, use the reverse Trendelenburg positioning. Be very liberal with oxygen in a pregnant patient even if their oxygen saturation is within normal limits. Hyperoxygenate before any attempts at airway or expected periods of apnea as pregnant patients do not have the reserve to tolerate hypoxia. Maintain the appropriate $PaCO_2$ for stage of pregnancy. In late pregnancy, normal $PaCO_2$ is 30 mm Hg (respiratory alkalosis of pregnancy); therefore, a $PaCO_2$ of 35 to 45 mmHg may indicate impending respiratory failure. Use continuous pulse oximetry and end-tidal CO_2 monitoring when able.

- C: Circulation and hemorrhage control

Asses for obvious signs of hemorrhage, including quick vaginal inspection, and examine any open wounds. Keep in mind that pregnant patients may not exhibit physical signs of hypovolemia until 35% to 45% of blood volume is lost.[9] The uterus lacks autoregulation; therefore, hemodynamic changes in blood volume are immediately reflected in the uterus and fetus. Fetal distress may be present before any signs of maternal hemodynamic compromise.[8]

- D: —Disability (neurologic assessment) and displacement of uterus

Assess for neurologic function including motor and sensation. If over 20 weeks and able, place patient in lateral positioning to displace the uterus. If unable to place in this position (unstable, cardiac arrest) then use manual pressure to displace the uterus laterally preventing IVC syndrome and aortic compression. Compression of the IVC reduces cardiac output and can exacerbate shock states and hypotension.

- E: Exposure and environmental control

Remove any remaining garments to allow for full inspection and examination, including vaginal examination during secondary survey. Heat the room or use Bair Huggers or other warming devices as needed to prevent hypothermia.

- F: (specific to pregnancy) Fetal monitoring

In the case of pregnant trauma patients greater than 20 weeks, apply continuous fetal monitoring and contact the appropriate service lines (OBGYN, neonatology, and MFM).

As the primary surveyor, it is important to move quickly but thoroughly through each step, stopping to address abnormalities found in each step before continuing on. With each subsequent intervention, the primary survey is then repeated from the start, again moving quickly through each step.[8]

Secondary survey (FGHI)

The secondary survey is completed after the primary survey and interventions are done. The secondary survey consists of a systematic head-to-toe examination and obtaining any available history or pertinent information.[8]

- F: (secondary) Full set of vital signs, focused assessment with sonography for trauma (FAST)

Obtain a full set of vital signs, including fetal monitoring. Perform a FAST examination to quickly assess for internal hemorrhage, keeping in mind that FAST may not be as accurate in a highly gravid patient.[10]

- G: Give comfort
  Medicate symptoms such as pain and nausea as able, avoiding heavy sedation and respiratory depression, especially in the pregnant trauma patient. The use of multimodal pain regimens can help alleviate pain and minimize opioid use.
- H: History and head to toe including vaginal examination

Obtain any pertinent and available medical history from patient, emergency medical services (EMS), or bystanders/family members. The SAMPLE pneumonic can be used to obtain history (**Table 1**). Complete a head-to-toe examination including a vaginal examination. The vaginal examination is used to quickly determine the presence of blood, amniotic fluid, or preterm labor. Repeated vaginal examinations should be avoided.[8]

Table 1 The SAMPLE pneumonic provides a quick tool for obtaining pertinent history	
	SAMPLE
S	Signs and symptoms
A	Allergies
M	Medications
P	Pertinent past medical and obstetrics, obstetrician (OB) history
L	Last oral intake
E	Events leading to current event

- I: Inspect posterior surface

With assistance, use a log-roll technique to turn patient and inspect the back for spinal step-off or tenderness. Inspect the posterior skin for abrasions or wounds, including entrance/exit wounds in the event of penetrating trauma. Finally, perform a digital rectal examination for rectal tone and presence of blood in the rectal vault.

Fetal–maternal hemorrhage (Kleihauer–Betke assay [KB] stain)

Whenever there is abdominal or multisystem trauma, anterior placenta, or uterine tenderness, the fetal–maternal hemorrhage should be suspected and evaluated. The Kleihauer–Betke assay (KB stain) will test for the presence of fetal red blood cells in the maternal system.[5] The KB stain is obtained through a maternal blood sample. A positive test indicates fetal–maternal hemorrhage. Another test, the flow cytometry test, has been shown to be superior to the KB stain.[5] Flow cytometry is a laboratory method to count and identify characteristics of the red blood cells in body fluids. Depending on resources and location, one of these tests for fetal-maternal hemorrhage should be considered in the pregnant trauma patient.

Isoimmunization and RhoGam

All pregnant women who are Rh negative with a positive KB stain should receive RH immune globulin (RhoGam) intramuscularly. To prevent isoimmunization, this should be administered within 72 hours of the injury. Usually, a 300-μg dose will protect against fetal blood cells in the maternal circulation. Should the patient not a have a positive KB stain, RhoGam should still be considered in a nonimmunized trauma patient. Even a very small amount of fetal blood in maternal circulation can lead to isoimmunization or DIC.

Radiology

Exposure to necessary radiologic procedures during trauma evaluation confers a risk of childhood cancer of approximately one in 1000 to one in 1,000,000 depending on the number and types of scans.[11] Ultrasound is noninvasive and not harmful to mother or fetus; therefore, it is used as a part of the secondary survey to assess for internal hemorrhage by performing a FAST examination. Plain radiographs also used to obtain chest and pelvis films during the secondary survey and can be used to evaluate for major thoracic and pelvic trauma.[8] In the event of severe obvious injuries or suspected thoracic and abdominal traumatic injuries, however, a CT scan is warranted.[8] Sakowicz and colleagues performed a retrospective cohort study of 119 pregnant patients evaluated for major trauma at two level-1 trauma centers between 2003 and 2019.[12] They evaluated different imaging techniques used on pregnant trauma patients including CT abdomen and pelvis (CTAP), FAST, and combinations of the two imaging modalities in detecting intra-abdominal hemorrhage and injury. Their study demonstrated that FAST alone is not as accurate in detecting intra-abdominal hemorrhage and injury in pregnant trauma patients and CTAP should be the preferred imaging technique if indicated.[12] Furthermore, the sensitivity for CT is 100% and specificity 54% to 56% and performs better than ultrasound at detecting clinical abruptions.[10]

MANAGEMENT
Mechanism of Injury

According to a systematic review by DeVito and colleagues, MVCs account for the majority of trauma in pregnancy.[13] Pregnancy changes the expected injury patterns due to alterations in anatomy and physiology. With MVCs, the injury patterns vary based on location of the patient in the vehicle, vehicle speed, proper use of restraints, and extenuating circumstances such as prolonged extrication, exposure to smoke or chemicals, or death in the vehicle. MVCs are commonly associated with blunt force trauma including head trauma, spinal trauma, thoracic and abdominal trauma, and orthopedic injuries. They are also associated with shear force (coup) and tensile force (contre-coup) injuries due to velocity.[8] Frequently in pregnancy, restraints such as shoulder and lap belts are not worn or are worn incorrectly, leading to a preventable cause of traumatic injury. The type of restraint system used affects the frequency of uterine rupture and fetal death.[8]

The next most common cause of injury in pregnancy is related to falls, assaults, and IPV. As with MVCs, falls, assaults, and IPV frequently result in blunt force injuries. With assaults and IPV, however, there is also the threat of penetrating trauma from the use of guns or knives. Seventeen percent of injured pregnant patients experience trauma inflicted by another person, and 60% of these patients experience repeated episodes of IPV.[8] Recognizing IPV is essential. Any suspicion of IPV should be documented and reported. Consider IPV when the following are present:

- Injuries that are not consistent with the story
- Suicide attempts or evidence of depression
- Self-abuse
- Frequent emergency department (ED) visits
- Substance abuse
- Self-blame for injuries
- Partner insistent on being present for interview, examination, and they are the only one speaking.

Blunt trauma
Blunt traumatic injuries can occur from direct and indirect force on the abdomen as a result of airbags, restraints, crush injuries, gravitational force, velocity, and direct blows. Owing to the anatomic changes that occur with pregnancy, especially late pregnancy, the injury patterns for blunt trauma change. Initially, the uterus lies within the pelvis; thus, abdominal injury patterns are similar to nonpregnant trauma patients with the exception of bony pelvic fractures. Bony pelvic fractures in early and very late pregnancy can be associated with uterine injury, placental abruption/rupture, and fetal injury. Late in pregnancy the fetal head descends into the pelvis, increasing risk of fetal cranial injuries with pelvic fractures.[8] The layering of the abdominal wall, uterine wall, and amniotic fluid provides a barrier for the most part for direct fetal injury. Indirect fetal injury may also occur from tensile and shear forces associated with rapid deceleration, high-level falls, or direct blows from objects. Utilization of restraint belts also contribute to blunt injury if worn incorrectly. Shearing and tensile forces can also cause

placental abruption, uterine wall rupture, and disruption of the vessels within the uterine wall leading to hemorrhage.

Penetrating trauma

From 20 weeks gestation onward, the uterus is somewhat protective of the abdominal organs related to penetrating trauma. Therefore, most of the injury patterns during this time will directly affect the uterus and/or fetus rather than the abdominal organs. Later in pregnancy, the bowels are displaced cephalad, so high abdominal penetrating wounds have a greater chance of causing hollow viscus injury than usual. As mentioned previously, FAST is useful but less sensitive/specific for hollow injury and bleeding in pregnant trauma patients; therefore, CTAP should still be used when indicated.[12]

Placental abruption

Placental abruption is a leading cause of fetal death particularly in cases of blunt abdominal trauma.[7] Within the muscular uterus, a rigid placenta can detach due to the shearing force of trauma from a blunt abdominal injury.[7] Placental abruption presents within the initial hours of the event to up to 24 hours later. The pregnant trauma victim should be monitored for at least 24 hours following an abdominal injury. Symptoms of placental abruption may include a rigid "board-like" abdomen or uterine tenderness, small frequent uterine contractions, vaginal bleeding, and nonreassuring fetal heart rate. Uterine contractions are the most significant indicator of placental abruption.[7]

Uterine rupture

Uterine rupture is a very rare occurrence; however, it is an important consideration in the pregnant trauma patient. Fetal mortality is 100% and maternal mortality is 10% when uterine rupture occurs.[5] The symptoms of uterine rupture may include intense abdominal pain, vaginal bleeding, palpation of fetal parts on the abdominal examination, nonreassuring fetal heart rate, and maternal hypovolemia. The immediate delivery of the fetus and hysterectomy or uterine repair is indicated.[5]

Preterm labor

Uterine assessment should be done on all pregnant patients with a fetal gestation greater than 22 weeks. This includes fundal assessment, palpation for uterine tenderness, and application of uterine monitoring for the presence of uterine contractions. In addition, sterile speculum examination should occur to check for rupture of membranes or pooling of fluid in the back of the vagina. If the membranes are intact and abruption has been ruled out, it is advisable to administer tocolytics such as indomethacin or nifedipine. The tocolytics allow time to administer corticosteroids to enhance lung maturity in the fetus should delivery occur. Betamethasone 12 mg intramuscularly for two doses given 12 hours apart is the general premedication for preterm labor. Finally, magnesium sulfate intravenously beginning with a 4-g bolus followed by 2 g per hour for 24 hours should be given for neuroprotection of the fetus if the pregnant patient is less than 32 weeks gestation and at risk of preterm labor.[7]

Fetal patient

Uterine artery perfusion depends on maternal mean arterial pressure as the uterus lacks autoregulation. If the pregnant trauma victim is hypotensive, there will be uterine hypoperfusion. In the case of fulminant maternal shock, there is uterine vasoconstriction resulting in uterine hypoperfusion and decreased oxygenation to the fetus. Fetal distress and hypoperfusion may occur before signs of maternal shock as a result of the physiologic changes of pregnancy and increased blood volume. Assessment of the fetal heart tracing may reveal bradycardia, tachycardia, decreased variability or the presence of late decelerations.

During trauma, the fetus is generally protected by the amniotic fluid, placenta, uterus, and abdominal soft tissue. Amniotic fluid serves as a buffer for force and absorbs and dissipates some force and decelerates projectiles. Fetal injuries most often occur during the third trimester due to the presence of a thin-walled uterus, less abdominal fluid, and engagement into the pelvis. If engagement has occurred, the fetus is at risk for fetal skull and brain injury due to impact from the maternal bony pelvis.

SPECIAL CONSIDERATIONS
Perimortem Cesarean Delivery

Should maternal cardiac arrest occur and the fetus is viable (>24 weeks), it is recommended to deliver the fetus within the first 5 minutes. In 1986, Katz originally proposed perimortem cesarean section by which emptying the uterus relieves the uteroplacental circuit and aortocaval compression, thereby increasing venous return and cardiac output in the patient with a 20-week fetus.[14] He was able to prove improved outcomes. This was further studied in 2005.[15] On the 4th minute of arrest with no return of spontaneous circulation, the physician should make the initial incision. Delivery should occur in the trauma bay rather than moving the patient to the operating room (OR) or delivery area.[14]

CLINICS CARE POINTS

- Placental vasculature is dilated and lacks autoregulation; therefore, any changes in maternal hemodynamics will reflect directly on the placental circulation and the fetus. Pregnant patients may lose up to 30% to 40% of blood volume before manifesting changes in hemodynamics. Fetal distress may be present when the mother has no hemodynamic abnormalities.

- Pregnant trauma patients lack reserve to tolerate hypoxia. Early and liberal oxygenation is indicated even in stable pregnant trauma patients. Hyperoxygenation and upright positioning should be used to prevent hypoxia during airway attempts. A normal $PaCO_2$ may indicate impending respiratory failure in a pregnant patient.

- When transporting and managing pregnant trauma patients, they should be placed in left lateral decubitus position to prevent inferior vena cava syndrome and hypotension. The log-roll technique or manual displacement of the uterus to the left may be used.

- The severity of maternal injuries determines maternal and fetal outcome. Initial resuscitation and treatment priorities remain the same as for the nonpregnant patient. The best initial treatment for the fetus is the provision of optimal resuscitation of the mother.

SUMMARY

Anatomic and physiologic changes occur during pregnancy that can influence the assessment and treatment of injured pregnant patients. The unique challenges of caring for the pregnant trauma patient can be overcome by using a systematic, organized method of assessment and resuscitation. A multidisciplinary team-based approach is essential to promote well-being of both mother and fetus.

REFERENCES

1. Sakamoto J, Michels C, Eisfelder B, et al. Trauma in pregnancy. Emer Med Clin 2019;37:317–38. https://doi.org/10.1016/j.emc.2019.01.009.

2. Huls CK, Detlefs C. Trauma in pregnancy. Semin Perin 2018;42:13–20. https://doi.org/10.1053/j.semperi.2017.11.004.

3. Mendez-Figueroa H, Dahlke JD, Vrees RA, et al. Trauma in pregnancy: an updated systematic review. Am Jour Ob Gyn 2013;209(1):1–10. https://doi.org/10.1016/j.ajog.2013.01.021.

4. Dalton S, Stamilio D, Sakowicz A, et al. Association between timing of major trauma in pregnancy and adverse outcomes related to placental dysfuncion. Am Jour Ob Gyn 2022;226(1):S533–4.

5. Cunningham F, Leveno KJ, Dashe JS, et al, editors. Williams Obstetrics. 26e. McGraw Hill; 2022.

6. Clark SL, Cotton DB, Lee W, et al. Central hemodynamic assessment of normal term pregnancy. Am Jour Ob Gyn 1989;161(6Pt1):1439–42. https://doi.org/10.1016/0002-9378(89)90900-9.

7. Greco PS, Day LJ, Pearlman MD. Guidance for evaluation and management of blunt abdominal trauma in pregnancy. Obst & Gyn 2022;134(6):1343–57. https://doi.org/10.1097/AOG.0000000000003585.

8. American College of Surgeons. Committee on trauma. Advanced trauma Life Support: Student course manual. 10th edition. Chicago: American College of Surgeons; 2018.

9. Wilkerson RG, Yuan S, Windsor TA. Trauma in pregnancy: a comprehensive overview. Trauma Rep 2020;21(3):1–15.

10. Jha P, Melendres G, Bijan B, et al. Trauma in pregnant women: assessing detection of post-traumatic placental abruption on contrast-enhanced CT versus ultrasound. Abd Radiol 2017;42:1062–7.

11. Wiles R, Hankinson B, Benbow E, et al. Making decisions about radiological imaging in pregnancy. BMJ 2022;377:e070486. https://doi.org/10.1136/bmj-2022-070486.

12. Sakowicz A, Dalton S, McPherson J, et al. Accuracy and utilization patterns of intra-abdominal imaging for major trauma in pregnancy. Am Jour Ob Gyn 2022;226(1):S195–6.

13. DeVito M, Capannolo G, Alameddine S, et al. Trauma in pregnancy clinical practice guidelines: a systematic review. The Jour of Mat-Fet & Neon Med 2022. https://doi.org/10.1080/14767058.2022.2078190.

14. Katz VL, Dotters DJ, Droegemueller W. Perimortem cesarean delivery. Obst and Gyn 1986;64(4):571–6.

15. Katz VL, Balderson K, Defreest M. Perimortem cesarean delivery: Were our assumptions correct? Am Jour Ob Gyn 2005;192:1916–21.

Impact of the Social Determinants of Health on Adult Trauma Outcomes

Quinn Lacey, PhD, RN, CCRN

KEYWORDS

- Social determinants of health • Trauma outcomes • Mortality • Disparities

KEY POINTS

- Disparities in trauma outcomes
- Race, socioeconomic status, and insurance status matter
- Increased trauma mortality rates among minorities

INTRODUCTION

Social determinants of health (SDOHs) have been well studied within the literature in the United States (US) but the effects of these determinants of health on patients with trauma have garnered less attention. The interaction between patients with SDOHs and patients with trauma requires clinicians caring for this population to view patients with trauma through a multifaceted lens. The purpose of this article will be to illuminate the drivers of trauma in the adult population and how the SDOHs and the health-care system come together to contribute to disparities in trauma outcomes.

Background

According to the Centers for Disease Control and Prevention (CDC), SDOHs are those social and economic conditions that influence the health of individuals.[1] The World Health Organization (WHO) implores the medical community and policymakers to implement health policies and guidelines based on SDOHs. By not accounting for SDOHs in caring for patients, health interventions may provide limited benefit.[2–4] Focusing on the determinants of health, Healthy People 2030 groups the SDOHs into 5 domains:[1]

1. Economic stability
2. Education access and quality

LSU Health-New Orleans, School of Nursing, 1900 Gravier Street, New Orleans, LA 70112, USA
E-mail address: qlace1@lsuhsc.edu

Crit Care Nurs Clin N Am 35 (2023) 223–233
https://doi.org/10.1016/j.cnc.2023.02.013
0899-5885/23/© 2023 Elsevier Inc. All rights reserved.

3. Health care access and quality
4. Neighborhood and built environment
5. Social and community context

Minority groups in America seem to experience higher mortality rates when it comes to trauma outcomes.[1,5] The effects of race/ethnicity, socioeconomic status (SES), and insurance on trauma mortality rates are ill-defined at best, throughout the literature. What the literature does reveal is that trauma is not experienced uniformly[6]; using a sample of 75,351 patients with spinal trauma the study found that the odds ratio for mortality in African American patients with trauma ($P = .0001$) was only second to the mortality rate of patients with trauma presenting in shock. Minorities, the poor, and the uninsured experience disproportionately different outcomes.[5,6] One would think that in today's society, where health care is increasingly under the watchful eye of the federal government as well as several agencies and carrying the banner of equal access for all that current research would reveal similar trauma outcome statistics for all American adults. Unfortunately, studies reveal data in which there is evidence that disparities in trauma outcomes are real.

Insurance status disparities in trauma outcomes among adults have spawned interest in how insurance status can influence trauma outcomes. A study by Downing and colleagues[7] concluded that mortality rates of trauma survivors on day 2 of admission differed by insurance status with the disparities becoming more pronounced throughout the hospital stay. Furthermore, Downing and colleagues[7] concluded that through subset analysis, by focusing on patients aged 19 to 30 years, they could mitigate the possibility that differences in comorbidities could cause insurance status disparity. It may be difficult to determine the cause of trauma outcome disparities among adult victims but 3 factors have been identified as domains for speculative decision-making: the patient, the hospital, and the timeliness of treatment.

Patients with trauma or family members of patients with trauma that have little or no insurance may have anxiety about making decisions about life-sustaining procedures for loved ones in face of their inability to pay.[8] Family members of uninsured trauma victims may be less likely to accept the continuation of heroic efforts given the presumed permanent disability or cost of continued care of the trauma survivor. Then, healthy uninsured trauma victims may leave against medical advice, increasing the disparity in the course of care. Hospitals often have policies that require additional forms to justify ordering expensive tests or medication for uninsured patients. At the provider level, unconscious motivation to withhold care cannot be ruled out.[9] There may also be altruistic motivation on the part of the provider in sparing uninsured families of patients with trauma the financial burden of seemingly unnecessary charges: reluctance to order tests or medications for uninsured trauma victims in the same timeframe as for insured victims may also increase mortality rates for uninsured trauma victims.[10]

Haider-Weygandt and colleagues,[9] conducting a meta-analysis, concluded that patients with trauma without insurance had higher mortality rates than patients with trauma with insurance ($P = .05$). Regional and national studies within the National Trauma Data Bank (NTDB) were consistent in illuminating higher mortality rates among uninsured patients with trauma.[9] Unconscious bias regarding insurance status and quality of care is difficult to examine. Timing to critical procedures after a traumatic accident is a much better gauge by which to evaluate disparities among insured and noninsured patients.

The time it takes for definitive treatment after a traumatic accident is crucial. Any delay in additional evaluations, diagnostic tests, or intrafacility transport may influence mortality rates among trauma victims. In a single-facility, retrospective study, looking at standardized treatment protocols following trauma activation of 1219 patients in which 65% were men, 56.8% were White, 11.2% African-American, and 7.8% were Asian or Pacific Islander, de Angelis and collegues[10] found no association between outcomes and the timing of diagnostic procedures and treatments posttrauma activation but there were associations between the severity of the injury and secondarily insurance status.

It is often difficult to separate associations between insurance status and race when examining disparities in trauma outcomes. Within the literature, there is an increasing body of research describing racial disparities in posttraumatic outcomes. Several adult trauma studies have described differences in outcomes based on insurance status. In a multiple logistic regression analysis from the NTDB (2001–2005), Haider and collegues[11] found that in reviewing 429,751 patients aged 18 to 64 years with Injury Severity Scores (ISS) of 9 or greater, African Americans and Hispanic patients with trauma had higher unadjusted mortality rates than White patients after trauma. Illustrates the independent influence of insurance status on the odds of death compared between Whites, African Americans, and Hispanics in the US.[11]

Postulating predictors of morbidity and mortality after spinal trauma in a national model, Schoenfield and colleagues[6] used a weighed sample of 75,351 patients from the National Sample Program of the NTDB to reveal increased mortality and decreased hospital length of stay (LOS), intensive care unit (ICU) stays, and ventilator time for patients without health insurance (**Table 1**). Several factors were investigated as possible influences on the effect of SDOHs on trauma outcomes. Patient-based factors such as medical comorbidities, age, attitudes toward the health-care system, and mitigating factors such as trauma mechanism, the severity of the injury, and hospital quality all pose credible avenues for investigation. Although increased mortality may inherently have been associated with decreased LOS, ICU stays, and ventilator time among patients without insurance, similar parallels were not observed in the African American and non-White groups.[11]

Insurance status can be said to fall under the domain of economic stability within the SDOHs. After all, it is typically our economic status that determines whether we carry health insurance ourselves or not. If SDOHs include conditions where we are born, age, grow, live, and work, then it can be argued that race should be included as an SDOH. Heffernan and colleagues,[12] in performing multivariable logistic and proportional hazard regression analyses on 3101 traumatic brain injury (TBI) patients, found that non-White patients and patients without insurance were significantly less likely to be placed in a rehabilitation center. Mortality was unaffected by race but increased in intoxicated patients, with the lowest mortality rates in patients with private insurance.[12]

RACIAL DISPARITIES

Racial disparities in emergency or trauma care seem to receive less attention than other disparities such as access to care among a variety of other contexts, giving rise to the first consensus conference on disparities in emergency health care in 2003. There is a substantial body of evidence of racial disparities in access to care for a variety of medical conditions.[13] Several studies provide indications that minorities are at higher risk of death after trauma than White patients, and cannot simply be explained away by controlling for insurance status, SES, or clinical characteristics.[14–18]

Receiving treatment at a level I or II trauma center can greatly increase survival in trauma outcomes. Governments and policymakers at all levels of our society have

Table 1
The influence of race/ethnicity and insurance status on mortality, complications, length of hospital stay, length of intensive care unit days, and ventilator time

Risk Factor	Mortality OR (95% CI), P-Value	Complications OR (95% CI), P-Value	Hospital Stay RC (SD), P-Value	ICU Days RC (SD), P-Value	Ventilator Days RC (SD), P-Value
Nonwhite	1.6 (1.1, 2.4), .20	1.0 (0.8, 1.3), .9	0.8 (60.3), .02	1.0 (60.6), .1	1.1 (60.6), .1
Black/African American	2.1 (1.25, 3.6), .005	0.8 (0.6, 1.2), .3	1.0 (60.5), .05	0.6 (60.7), .4	-0.0 (60.8), 1.0
Insurance					
Government	0.5 (0.2, 1.4), .07	0.9 (0.6, 1.4), .8	0.7 (61.0), .5	-0.4 (60.9), .7	0.9 (61.5), .6
Medicare and Medicaid	1.15 (1.0, 1.4), .76	1.1 (0.9, 1.2), .07	1.3 (60.5), .01	1.3 (61.3), .3	3.5 (61.1), .002
None	2.0 (1.5, 2.7), .002	0.9 (0.7, 1.2), .9	-1.0 (60.35), .006	-1.6 (60.6), .006	-1.95 (60.9), .03
Other	2.6 (1.1, 5.8), .02	0.9 (0.55, 1.4), .8	0.4 (60.4), .3	0.2 (60.75), .75	0.1 (61.0), .9
Workers' compensation	0.6 (0.3, 1.2), .04	0.8 (0.6, 1.1), .4	-0.0 (60.4), 1.0	-0.1 (60.95), .9	-1.6 (61.1), .1

Statistically, significant P values are highlighted in bold.

Abbreviations: 95% CI, 95% confidence interval; ICU, intensive care unit; OR, odds ratio; RC, regression coefficient; SD, standard deviation.

From Schoenfeld AJ, Belmont PJ Jr, See AA, Bader JO, Bono CM. Patient demographics, insurance status, race, and ethnicity as predictors of morbidity and mortality after spine trauma: a study using the National Trauma Data Bank. Spine J. 2013;13(12):1766-1773. https://doi.org/10.1016/j.spinee.2013.03.024.

aimed to standardize trauma systems around the country. Despite these efforts, racial disparities in trauma outcomes still persist and cannot be explained by adjusting for comorbidities and injury characteristics. There is evidence that minorities living in rural communities, particularly African Americans and Latinos, have increased trauma mortality rates, leading some researchers to suspect that the problem may exist at the system level. Alber and colleagues[18] found that African Americans and Latinos are undertriaged to the appropriate level of trauma centers. African American communities and other vulnerable populations were also found to be disproportionately affected by declining access to trauma centers due to hospital closures in urban areas.[19]

According to the CDC, where one lives and their economic status can influence the health of individuals. Previous studies examining geographic access to trauma care found differences between urban and rural regions around the country.[20] Crandall and colleagues[21] used the term trauma desert to describe regions greater than 8 miles from the nearest trauma center. Using census tract data, Tung examined 3 geographic trauma deserts and access to trauma care in 3 major cities across America, Los Angeles (LA), CA, Chicago, Illinois, and New York City (NYC). The Tung study concluded that census tracts within LA ($P < .01$) and Chicago ($P < .001$), where the majority of the population was African Americans were consistently more likely to be located in trauma deserts than white census tracts.[20] Although there were no significant racial/ethnic disparities in NYC, regarding census tract data and trauma deserts, a residual direct effect was observed after adjusting for poverty and race-poverty interaction effects ($P < .01$).[20] Hispanic/Latino majority census tracts within the study were less likely to be in trauma deserts in LA ($P < .001$) and NYC ($P < .001$) but slightly more likely in Chicago ($P < .001$).

There has been extensive research providing evidence that African Americans and Latinos suffer higher mortality rates than Whites after traumatic motor vehicle crashes (MVCs).[22–24] In a study examining traumatic MVC survival by race, Haskin[15] further examined 3 components of traumatic MVC survival by race: overall survival, survival to reach a hospital, and survival among those hospitalized. Using national, publicly available data from the National Automotive Sampling System Crashworthiness Data System between 2000 and 2008, Haskins[15] found that race was not significantly associated with overall survival after a traumatic MVC, and that African Americans and Latinos were equally likely to survive traumatic MVCs but African Americans treated at hospitals after a traumatic MVC were 50% less likely to survive after 30 days of hospitalization compared with White patients (OR = 0.50, 95% CI: 0.33, 0.76).

Using the State Inpatient database for Michigan and all trauma-related admissions between 2006 and 2014 in the Detroit metropolitan area (N = 407,553), a study by Loberg and colleagues[25] examined the relationships between race, socioeconomic background, and in-hospital trauma mortality. Compared with other groups in the study, African Americans were 20% more likely to die from traumatic injuries than White patients. When considering the trauma types, the disparity could still not be statistically explained, and although higher mortality trauma mechanisms were observed in the African American patients with trauma, race was still significantly associated with trauma mortality ($P < .001$). Loberg[25] also found that there were associations between SES and insurance status where a 1% increase in poverty rate increased mortality in patients with trauma by 1%.

Socioeconomic Status

It is well accepted that the broad concept of SES plays a role in patients' morbidity and mortality.[26–28] Exploring how SES influenced patients aged 65 years and older, Romanowski and colleagues[29] retrospectively pooled data from 3 verified burn centers between 2004 and 2014 by race, age, gender, total body surface area (%TBSA) burned, LOS, and LOS burned per %TBSA. Using the US census to compile data on race, poverty, and educational levels within a community, race was not a predictor of mortality in elderly patients aged 65 years and older but SES independently predicted LOS as well as discharge to a skilled nursing facility ($P = .001$).[29] Studying the effect of SES on burn victim outcomes, Bedri and colleagues,[30] using a retrospective review of 135,680 patients from the National Burn Repository (version 8, 2002–2011), found that even though minority groups, consistent with existing literature, were found to have greater numbers of uninsured patients compared with White patients, SES had no significant association with mortality in respect to severe burn outcomes.[30]

Examining associations between trauma burn patients and SES, Doctor[31] explored the socioeconomic impact of postburn patients with TBSA greater than 15% between 2005 and 2012 and found that those in low-socioeconomic groups had 5 times the odds of having graft loss than those in high-socioeconomic groups.[31] The author goes on to suggest that the effect of comorbidities such as obesity, smoking, and diabetes within the low-socioeconomic population may explain the increased risk of graft loss.[31] Disparities in trauma outcomes related to SES are not isolated to America but are a global phenomenon. Abedzadeh-Kalahroudi[32] examined 600 patients with trauma in Kashan, Iran, using demographic and trauma-related questionnaires, a socioeconomic assessment scale, the hospital care index, and the WHO Disability Assessment Schedule-II tool and concluded that patients with low SES were at greater risk for low-level care and subsequent higher trauma mortality.[32] Haines and colleagues[33] used a retrospective cohort of 106,708 TBI procedures from the NTDB (2012–2015) and found that individuals with low SES were more likely to be afflicted by TBI than those with high SES. In their study, they also found disparities in LOS among African Americans, Latinos, and Medicaid patients throughout the spectrum of severity. What the study concluded was that minorities and the uninsured with TBI had the greatest disparities in treatment and outcomes.[33]

THE ENVIRONMENT

As one of the SDOHs, an individual's environment plays a major role in the health of that individual.[34] Trauma systems were created to improve the mortality rates of patients by providing specialty care but all trauma systems are not created equally. Trauma systems that service large geographic areas, particularly rural areas, have higher mortality rates in rural populations.[35,36] A major goal for trauma systems is getting the patient to the appropriate place at the right time and including hospitals with varying levels of care provision and resources.[37] In an integrative literature review, Morgan and Calleja[37] found that there were several challenges to providing trauma care to patients in rural communities.

In examining factors that were associated with the remoteness of a community affecting trauma outcomes, Morgan and Calleja[37] used an integrative literature review and discovered that even the term remote was not easily defined across studies. Different countries had different interpretations of what remote meant. Although one study described remoteness as having very restricted access to goods, services, and social interaction, another study used the Accessibility/Remotes Index of Australia scoring system where remote is a score of 5.92 to less than 10.53: based on averaging road distance to several surrounding towns.[38] Having limited access to services and resources in rural settings underscores another challenge for patients with trauma.[39] Other challenges observed where the environment is a factor in delays is in locating patients with trauma due to not remoteness or distance of the environment but in accessing difficult terrain in reaching victims. Research from Australia noted that as the risk of death increased with remoteness ($P < .001$),[40] the majority of deaths occurred prehospital,[41–43] suggesting that the "golden hour" in trauma care may be irrelevant because it pertains to remote or rural settings.[44] Simon, and colleagues[42] in studying prehospital time of arrival of patients with trauma in mountainous areas compared with those in urban and suburban areas found that trauma victims presenting in mountainous areas presented with different injury mechanisms, longer prehospital times, and higher frequency of helicopter emergency medical services dispatch. Mountain activities have become more popular over the years with increasing access to mountainous environments. Falls were the major mechanism of injury in the mountains, and there were no significant differences in mean ages found in the study.[42] The notion that mountain trauma victims are nearly always young might be a thing of the past.

The impact of our environment can have a major influence on our health and is considered an SDOH.[34] Examining geographic areas within minority communities, Tung and colleagues[20] observations of so-called trauma deserts within communities of color have real-life ramifications for those suffering traumatic injuries within these areas. All-terrain vehicles (ATVs) and dirt bikes (DB) being ridden on urban city streets have become popular among young adults in many urban cities. This popularity is only exacerbated by social media highlighting this activity among viewers.

Because riding ATVs or DBs on city streets is illegal in many states, often these riders use speed to stay one step ahead of law enforcement, maneuvering around cars and pedestrians.[45] Butts and colleagues[46] conducted a 12-year-long study into injury patterns, morbidity, and mortality associated with urban off-road vehicle (UORV) crashes and hypothesized that UORV crashes would differ in injury patterns from rural off-road vehicle (RORV) crashes. After collecting data, there was no association found between helmet use and TBI in either the UORV or RORV crashes but when Abbreviated Injury Scale scores were examined, the UORV scores were significantly higher than those of the RORV riders (**Table 2**).[46] The UORV group presented with lower Glasgow Coma Scores ($P < .05$) and higher ISS than RORV riders.[46]

Table 2
Abbreviated Injury Scale head for urban off-road recreational vehicles and rural off-road recreational vehicles

AIS Head Scores	Urban (%); $n = 200$	Rural (%); $n = 258$	P
AIS head (helmeted)			
0–1	22.5	50	<0.0001
2	9.5	12.8	0.0552
≥3	8	8.1	0.4125
AIS head (unhelmeted)			
0–1	36	17.4	<0.0001
2	10.5	6.6	0.5172
≥3	13.5	5	0.0304

Abbreviation: AIS, Abbreviated Injury Scale.
From Butts CA, Gonzalez R, Nguyen L, et al. Twelve-Year Review of Urban versus Rural Off-road Vehicle Injuries at a Level 1 Trauma Center. J Surg Res. 2019;233:331-334. https://doi.org/10.1016/j.jss.2018.07.061.

SOCIAL AND COMMUNITY CONTEXT

Whether or not we choose to wear a helmet when riding ATVs or DBs can often be influenced by one's associations with friends and whether or not it is what our peers or associates are doing within a group. Social and community context is another SDOH according to Health People 2030.[34] The repercussions of such a decision not to wear a helmet can have devastating results on trauma outcomes. For example, a study examining traumatic injury, mortality rates, and insurance status of ATV crash victims found that riders and passengers of ATVs who chose not to wear helmets not only sustained more traumatic injuries than helmeted riders ($P < .0001$) but those helmeted riders were also found more often to have personal insurance,[47] bringing again into question the role of SES and trauma outcomes. Further research is needed to perhaps examine the reasons why individuals choose not to wear helmets.

SUMMARY

Where we live, work, socialize, and access our health care influences our well-being and health. Trauma mortality rates are affected by race, SES, and insurance status yet many of these factors are ill-defined in the literature, and just how they affect trauma outcomes is unclear. Trauma is not experienced uniformly within society with minorities experiencing higher mortality rates and poorer outcomes. Our activities, whether influenced by our affinities with others or our neighborhoods, can contribute to higher severity scores in traumatic injuries, possibly leading to poorer trauma outcomes. Although there seems to be an increase in research on race and SES because they intersect with trauma outcomes, more research may be needed to possibly examine how an individual's culture influences trauma outcomes.

CLINICS CARE POINTS

- Social-economic status, race, and ethnicity are intimately intertwined.
- Make an effort to discuss with patients their social issues in regards to their health.
- Advocate for emergency service systems integration at the local and regional levels across all communities, urban and rural.
- Future research on insurance status and trauma outcomes should focus on specific types and not just whether a patient is covered or not.

REFERENCES

1. U.S department of health and human services. Social determinants of health. Office of Disease prevention and health. 2021. Available at: https://health.gov/healthypeople/priority-areas/social-determinants-health. Accessed July 12, 2022.
2. Phelos H, Kass N, Deeb A, et al. Social determinants of health and patient-level mortality prediction after trauma. Journal of Trauma and Acute Care Surgery 2022;92(2):287–95.
3. Greene WR, Oyetunji TA, Bowers U, et al. Insurance status is a potent predictor of outcomes in both blunt and penetrating trauma. Am J Surg 2010;199(4):554–7.
4. Arthur M, Hedges JR, Newgard CD, et al. Racial disparities in mortality among adults hospitalized after injury. Med Care 2008;46(2):192–9.

5. Mikhail JN, Nemeth LS, Mueller M, et al. The social determinants of trauma: a trauma disparities scoping review and framework. J Trauma Nurs 2018;25(5): 266–81.

6. Schoenfeld AJ, Belmont PJ Jr, See AA, et al. Patient demographics, insurance status, race, and ethnicity as predictors of morbidity and mortality after spine trauma: a study using the National Trauma Data Bank. Spine J 2013;13(12): 1766–73.

7. Downing SR, Oyetunji TA, Greene WR, et al. The impact of insurance status on actuarial survival in hospitalized trauma patients: when do they die? J Trauma 2011;70(1):130–5 [published correction appears in J Trauma. 2011 Feb;70(2): 525. Cornwell, Edward E 3rd [added]].

8. Chapman EN, Kaatz A, Carnes M. Physicians and implicit bias: how doctors may unwittingly perpetuate health care disparities. J Gen Intern Med 2013;28(11): 1504–10.

9. Haider AH, Weygandt PL, Bentley JM, et al. Disparities in trauma care and outcomes in the United States: a systematic review and meta-analysis. J Trauma Acute Care Surg 2013;74(5):1195–205.

10. de Angelis P, Kaufman EJ, Barie PS, et al. Disparities in insurance status are associated with outcomes but not timing of trauma care. J Surg Res 2022;273: 233–46.

11. Haider AH, Chang DC, Efron DT, et al. Race and insurance status as risk factors for trauma mortality. Arch Surg 2008;143(10):945–9.

12. Heffernan DS, Vera RM, Monaghan SF, et al. Impact of socioethnic factors on outcomes following traumatic brain injury. J Trauma 2011;70(3):527–34.

13. Institute of Medicine (US). Committee on understanding and eliminating racial and ethnic disparities in health care. In: Smedley BD, Stith AY, Nelson AR, editors. Unequal treatment: confronting racial and ethnic disparities in health care. Washington (DC): National Academies Press (US); 2003.

14. Arthur M, Hedges JR, Newgard CD, et al. Racial disparities in mortality among adults hospitalized after injury. Med Care 2008;46(2):192–9.

15. Haskins AE, Clark DE, Travis LL. Racial disparities in survival among injured drivers. Am J Epidemiol 2013;177(5):380–7.

16. Bazarian JJ, Pope C, McClung J, et al. Ethnic and racial disparities in emergency department care for mild traumatic brain injury. Acad Emerg Med 2003;10(11): 1209–17.

17. Arango-Lasprilla JC, Kreutzer JS. Racial and ethnic disparities in functional, psychosocial, and neurobehavioral outcomes after brain injury. J Head Trauma Rehabil 2010;25(2):128–36.

18. Alber DA, Dalton MK, Uribe-Leitz T, et al. A multistate study of race and ethnic disparities in access to trauma care. J Surg Res 2021;257:486–92.

19. Holst JA, Perman SM, Capp R, et al. Undertriage of trauma-related deaths in U.S. Emergency departments. West. J Emerg Med 2016;17(3):315–23.

20. Tung EL, Hampton DA, Kolak M, et al. Race/ethnicity and geographic access to urban trauma care. JAMA Netw Open 2019;2(3):e190138.

21. Crandall M, Sharp D, Unger E, et al. Trauma deserts: distance from a trauma center, transport times, and mortality from gunshot wounds in Chicago. Am J Public Health 2013;103(6):1103–9.

22. Baker SP, Braver ER, Chen LH, et al. Motor vehicle occupant deaths among Hispanic and black children and teenagers. Arch Pediatr Adolesc Med 1998; 152(12):1209–12.

23. Braver ER. Race, Hispanic origin, and socioeconomic status in relation to motor vehicle occupant death rates and risk factors among adults. Accid Anal Prev 2003;35(3):295–309.

24. Harper JS, Marine WM, Garrett CJ, et al. Motor vehicle crash fatalities: a comparison of Hispanic and non-Hispanic motorists in Colorado. Ann Emerg Med 2000; 36(6):589–96.

25. Loberg JA, Hayward RD, Fessler M, et al. Associations of race, mechanism of injury, and neighborhood poverty with in-hospital mortality from trauma: a population-based study in the Detroit metropolitan area. Medicine (Baltim) 2018;97(39):e12606.

26. Kousiouris P, Klavdianou O, Douglas KAA, et al. Role of socioeconomic status (SES) in globe injuries: a review. Clin Ophthalmol 2022;16:25–31.

27. Bagher A, Andersson L, Wingren CJ, et al. Socio-economic status and major trauma in a Scandinavian urban city: a population-based case-control study. Scand J Public Health 2016;44(2):217–23.

28. Warren JR, Hernandez EM. Did socioeconomic inequalities in morbidity and mortality change in the United States over the course of the twentieth century? J Health Soc Behav 2007;48(4):335–51.

29. Romanowski KS, Zhou Y, Ten Eyck P, et al. Racial and socioeconomic differences affect outcomes in elderly burn patients. Burns 2021;47(5):1177–82.

30. Bedri H, Romanowski KS, Liao J, et al. A national study of the effect of race, socioeconomic status, and gender on burn outcomes. J Burn Care Res 2017;38(3): 161–8.

31. Doctor N, Yang S, Maerzacker S, et al. Socioeconomic status and outcomes after burn injury. J Burn Care Res 2016;37(1):e56–62.

32. Abedzadeh-Kalahroudi M, Razi E, Sehat M. The relationship between socioeconomic status and trauma outcomes. J Public Health 2018;40(4):e431–9.

33. Haines KL, Nguyen BP, Vatsaas C, et al. Socioeconomic status affects outcomes after severity-stratified traumatic brain injury. J Surg Res 2019;235:131–40.

34. U.S department of health and human services. Social determinants of health. Office of Disease prevention and health; 2021. Available at: https://health.gov/healthypeople/priority-areas/social-determinants-health. Accessed July 12, 2022.

35. National healthcare quality and disparities report: chartbook on rural healthcare. Rockville (MD): Agency for Healthcare Research and Quality (US); 2021.

36. Kristiansen T, Lossius HM, Rehn M, et al. Epidemiology of trauma: a population-based study of geographical risk factors for injury deaths in the working-age population of Norway. Injury 2014;45(1):23–30.

37. Morgan JM, Calleja P. Emergency trauma care in rural and remote settings: challenges and patient outcomes. Int Emerg Nurs 2020;51:100880.

38. Queensland Government. Accessibility/remoteness index of Australia: Queensland government statistician's office. Queensland Government Statitician's Office. Published 2019. Available at: https://www.qgso.qld.gov.au/about-statistics/statistical-standards-classifications/accessibility-remoteness-index-australia. Accessed July 23, 2022.

39. Rauch S, Dal Cappello T, Strapazzon G, et al. Pre-hospital times and clinical characteristics of severe trauma patients: a comparison between mountain and urban/suburban areas. Am J Emerg Med 2018;36(10):1749–53.

40. Fatovich DM, Phillips M, Langford SA, et al. A comparison of metropolitan vs rural major trauma in Western Australia. Resuscitation 2011;82(7):886–90.

41. Bakke HK, Wisborg T. Rural high north: a high rate of fatal injury and prehospital death. World J Surg 2011;35(7):1615–20.

42. Simons R, Brasher P, Taulu T, et al. A population-based analysis of injury-related deaths and access to trauma care in rural-remote Northwest British Columbia. J Trauma 2010;69(1):11–9.
43. Raatiniemi L, Steinvik T, Liisanantti J, et al. Fatal injuries in rural and urban areas in northern Finland: a 5-year retrospective study. Acta Anaesthesiol Scand 2016; 60(5):668–76.
44. Fatovich DM, Phillips M, Jacobs IG, et al. Major trauma patients transferred from rural and remote western Australia by the royal flying doctor service. J Trauma 2011;71(6):1816–20.
45. Nathan L., Riding with the 12 o'clock boys; the New York Times. Published 2013. Available at: http://www.nytimes.com/2013/12/03/opinion/riding-with-the-12-oclock-boys.html. Accessed July 22, 2022.
46. Butts CA, Gonzalez R, Nguyen L, et al. Twelve-year review of urban versus rural off-road vehicle injuries at a level 1 trauma center. J Surg Res 2019;233:331–4.
47. Merrigan TL, Wall PL, Smith HL, et al. The burden of unhelmeted and uninsured ATV drivers and passengers. Traffic Inj Prev 2011;12(3):251–5.

Using Principles of Therapeutic Communication to Enhance Trauma-Informed Care in the Critical Care Setting to Promote Positive Encounters

Liv Dinoso, DNP, PMHNP-BC, FNP-C, CNE[a],*,
Colette Baudoin, PhD (c), MSN, RN, CNE, OCN[b]

KEYWORDS

- Trauma-informed communication • Trauma-informed care/approach
- Therapeutic communication • Intensive care setting

KEY POINTS

- Intensive care settings are wrought with patients and families experiencing physical and psychological trauma. This setting can precipitate stressful situations that can cause acute trauma reactions.
- Trauma-informed care in the critical care setting is therapeutic and promotes healthy communication among health-care workers, patients, and their loved ones.
- Trauma-informed communication is recommended to promote positive patient outcomes and increase the critical care nurse's self-awareness of verbal and nonverbal therapeutic communication.

INTRODUCTION

The Substance Abuse and Mental Health Services Administration defines trauma as "an event or circumstance resulting in physical harm, emotional harm, and/or life-threatening harm," which has "lasting adverse effects on the individual's mental health, physical health, emotional health, social well-being, and/or spiritual well-being."[1] Traumatic events include natural disasters, war, violence, assault, abuse, accidents, the death of a loved one, bullying, discrimination, and witnessing these events.[2] In the United States, approximately 1 in 4 children will have suffered a traumatic event

---

[a] School of Nursing, Louisiana State University Health Sciences Center New Orleans, 1900 Gravier Street, #331, New Orleans, LA 70112, USA; [b] School of Nursing, Louisiana State University Health Sciences Center New Orleans, 1900 Gravier Street, #417, New Orleans, LA 70112, USA
* Corresponding author.
E-mail address: ldinos@lsuhsc.edu

Crit Care Nurs Clin N Am 35 (2023) 235–246
https://doi.org/10.1016/j.cnc.2023.02.014
0899-5885/23/© 2023 Elsevier Inc. All rights reserved.

by adulthood,[2] and between 62% and 90% of Americans will have experienced trauma as an adult.[3] Although the evidence of trauma may be present in the acute care setting in specific patient populations, past traumatic events can influence patients, caregivers, and health-care professionals alike. Recognizing this possibility in ourselves, as well as those we care for, can enhance the understanding of therapeutic care provided and the need to develop therapeutic communication to minimize the risk of confrontational interactions between staff and patients. Communication techniques used while collaborating with patients and families in this acute traumatic setting have the ability to create a setting in which situations can become emotionally charged. As health-care providers, recognizing the possibility of preexisting traumatic occurrences leading to the emotional changes seen in families and patients enables the development of therapeutic, trauma-informed care for the patient and family.

Each patient will experience, respond to, and process trauma uniquely. Trauma-informed communication (TIC) is an approach by health-care providers to mitigate the adverse effects of trauma in these patients.[4] TIC is embedded in trauma-informed care, and TIC is a skill that nurses can use to successfully engage with trauma survivors. TIC includes recognition of the possible existence of trauma-causing stress hormones to be released. The surge of adrenaline and cortisol physiologically influence the reaction of the person to the traumatic event confronting them. Past exposure to adverse childhood experiences (ACEs) and other past traumatic events can affect the reaction of the person to a new perceived threat to homeostasis in the form of a current trauma. Considering the preexisting mediating factors that may be present in the patient and family's past, health-care workers need to use communication built on active listening, respect, self-awareness, and relaxed body language to build a healthy working relationship with patients and families built on trust.[5]

DISCUSSION

Shortly after experiencing a trauma, patients will commonly show emotional symptoms such as anger, shame, sadness, fear, shock, hopelessness, denial, disbelief, confusion, irritability, anxiety, numbness, and/or mood swings. Patients can also exhibit emotional dysregulation leading to self-defeating behaviors such as substance use or self-injurious behaviors. Trauma can also cause dissociation or emotional withdrawal. It is also possible for the patient to have fragmented or missing memories of the event or to show distrust of the health-care staff.[6] The trauma may be acutely experienced in the intensive care setting, or may have occurred months or years earlier, creating an emotional imprint that affects a person as new traumas occur. Remembering these possible symptoms is essential in planning for care and creating TIC to facilitate effective coping. Important nursing interventions for a patient with psychological trauma include identifying and understanding the patient's response to the traumatic event and using TIC skills to create a safe space for the patient. This will help increase patient engagement and foster autonomy.

As reported by Beattie and colleagues, "a gap remains in understanding what has happened to clients that perpetrate violence, and the link between adverse childhood experiences (ACE), the neuroscience of threat, and trauma-informed care."[7] Themes developed at the conclusion of this qualitative study included "client stress and trauma, previous client trauma, the impact of care provision on the client and trauma-informed care."[7] Although this study took place in an emergency room setting, the risk factors for inappropriate reactivity and potential workplace violence could easily be compared with the stressors and traumas seen in the intensive care unit of the hospital as well. The acute, critical nature of the medical conditions of this population could bring forward memories of previous traumas and, in fact, could be similar to past traumas experienced resulting in a resurgence of the emotional turmoil felt in earlier traumatic occurrences. Additionally, the stressors of simply being in the intensive care unit have the potential for recall of posttraumatic situations. Creating a therapeutic milieu in which trauma-informed care is provided can assist in mediating the psychological and physical reactions of patients and families.[7]

This potential for inappropriate reactivity can be seen not just in the adult intensive care setting as noted in a reported case study by Hubbard and colleagues in the NICU setting with a neonate nearing the end of life.[8] As noted in this situation, clinicians need to work to recognize, accept, and understand the impact these chronic, past stressors can have on current traumas.

The need to accept and recognize the chronic stress experienced by many of the families of these patients should be recognized by clinicians needing to work. Hubbard and colleagues discussed 6 pillars or principles of trauma-informed care needing to be considered when caring for any patient but particularly those in acutely stressful or traumatic situations (**Box 1**). These pillars were noted to be developed and addressed during multidisciplinary meetings to discuss the provision of futile care in this situation and included cultural, historical, and gender issues, empowerment, voice and choice for parents and staff, collaboration and mutuality, peer support, trustworthiness and transparency, and physical and psychological safety for parents and staff.[8] The nurse should

---

Box 1
Six pillars of trauma-informed care

Safety
- Ensure the patient's emotional and physical safety
- Assess for traumatic triggers
- Create a plan to address patient's triggers
- Promote a daily routine
- Decrease stimuli and maintain a peaceful milieu

Trust
- Practice transparency and genuineness
- Ensure consistency and appropriate boundaries
- Take responsibility

Choice
- As safely as possible, allow patient autonomy
- Address and accept the patient's preferences
- Help the patient determine own goals and priorities

Collaboration
- Share power and expectations
- Collaborate on patient goals and priorities
- Support the patient emotionally

Empowerment
- Prioritize patient education and knowledge
- Teach and build patient skills
- Focus on patient's strengths
- Promote grit and resiliency

Cultural humility
- Be aware of one's own beliefs, values, and practices
- Transcend biases and stereotypes
- Advocate for the patient's cultural needs
- Obtain cultural knowledge
- Show cultural desire and genuine concern

be able to recognize the vulnerability of families and caregivers and base nursing care on these 6 pillars of trauma-informed care while using TIC skills. The underpinnings of this study showed the complexity of the unspoken traumas that frequently burden patients and families. Attempts to manage the turmoil caused by these traumas can result in miscommunication and unpleasant encounters for the staff and those being care for alike. Antonucci and colleagues recognized the need to communicate with patients and families effectively and empathetically.[9] Yet, time constraints frequently prevent this from occurring and may result in miscommunication.

The goals of TIC are rooted in trauma-informed care's core principles of safety, trustworthiness and transparency, peer support, collaboration, empowerment, humility and responsiveness, and therapeutic communication.[10] Throughout the patient's care, TIC aims to provide a physically and psychologically safe space where both parties can collaborate and support shared decision-making to minimize power differences. TIC strives for mutual trust to meet patient goals, allow for care providers to recognize their own biases and stereotypes, and offer unique, culturally responsive care to the patient.

RECOMMENDATIONS

Therapeutic communication is embedded in TIC, and many recommendations stem from good sense, sound judgment, and respect for others. **Box 2** summarizes key principles in therapeutic communication that can be used to communicate with critical care patients. In the critical care setting, it would be prudent to first introduce yourself to patients and loved ones using your name and role, and then explain to the patient what you plan to do.[11] A simple introduction builds trust, alleviates fear, and clarifies any confusion. Not doing so may promote distrust, alienation, and fear in the patient. Demonstrating the desire to not just be task focused but to recognize the importance of the patient and family as well as the desire to understand the preferences of the patient and family when possible. Even in the busiest of situations, the ability of the nurse or health-care team to show intent to keep the family and patient aware of the situation has the potential to prevent inappropriate reactivity.

Second, the nurse should maintain the patient's privacy in a private environment. This means speaking with the patient alone first if possible and asking if they prefer to be alone or accompanied while you speak with them. The patient's environment should be safe and free from unwanted visitors and intrusion.[11] The patient should also be educated on legal considerations and policies of the organization in terms of health information and privacy. This establishes safety, promotes trust and transparency, and shows consideration of the patient's needs. Recognizing the different dynamics of any given situation becomes essential to the health-care provider managing the patient in this situation. In cases when the patient cannot speak for themselves, the family dynamics and the past traumas they have experienced both individually and as a family can quickly escalate inappropriately. Of utmost importance becomes the responsibility of the health-care provider to recognize the need for assistance in managing the situation while providing optimum care for the patient.

From the start of any encounter, the nurse should show awareness of their own kinetic communication composed of gestures. Gestures should be smooth and unobtrusive, and body movement should remain relaxed and unhurried to the extent possible. Excess energy in the nurse can manifest as fidgeting, tapping, scratching, hair-twirling, pen-clicking, foot tapping, or frequent phone checking.[12] These gestures imply the nurse is uneasy, anxious, bored, or inattentive. Excessive gesturing by the nurse could be overstimulating, distracting, or annoying to the patient. The same holds

Box 2

Key recommendations for using therapeutic communication in trauma-informed care

Introduction
- Introduce yourself to patient and others in the room using name and role[11]
- Explain what you are doing or what you are about to do[11]

Maintain privacy
- Ask to speak to the patient alone first
- Ask the patient if they prefer to be alone or accompanied during your care
- Keep the patient's environment safe and free from unwanted intrusion[11]
- Educate the patient on health information and policies on privacy

Kinetic communication
- Show awareness of one's own body and gestures
- Gestures are smooth and unobtrusive[12]
- Body movement is unhurried and relaxed
- Avoid tapping, fidgeting, hair-twirling, pen-clicking, and phone-checking[12]
- Maintain an erect posture slightly leaning toward the patient[12]
- Keep arms uncrossed by the side of the body

Facial expression
- Keep facial expressions neutral or congruent to conversation.
- Can show interest and kindness smiling with relaxed face muscles and slightly raised eyebrows[13]
- Avoid exaggerated facial expressions
- Eye contact is direct and culturally responsive

Active listening
- Look at the patient directly when talking
- Clear own thoughts of distractions
- Avoid planning out answers
- Intermittently nod to signal attentiveness[12]
- Use techniques such as reflection, seeking clarification, restating, and paraphrasing

Body proxemics
- Maintain distance during communication that is at the patient's comfort level
- Professional distance while with the patient is appropriate. This includes being an arm's length away from the patient[12]
- Try to meet the patient at the patient's level, especially if the patient is sitting or in bed[16]

Haptics
- Use therapeutic touch carefully and only after obtaining permission from the patient first[15]

Paralinguistic communication
- Speak in a softer volume, slower pace, and sincere intonation[15]

Patient-centered mindset
- Speak plainly, honestly, and straightforwardly[15]
- Use plain language that the patient can understand at the patient's education level.

Cultural humility
- Self-evaluate own beliefs
- Be humble
- Be willing to adapt to changes
- Promote respect and appreciation for each unique patient
- Ask about preferred pronouns
- Identify Safe Zone training opportunities to care for LGBTQ + patients
- Offer an interpreter if appropriate
- Self-critique own preconceived opinions, biases, and stereotypes

Therapeutic silence
- Use silence to serve a purpose
- Silence should be meaningful, reflective, and contemplative

for body movement since frequent body changes can imply boredom or lack of interest and caring. Smooth gestures and body movements show the nurse is confident and relaxed.

When sitting, the nurse should also maintain an erect posture that is slightly leaning toward the patient, and body stance should be open with arms uncrossed at the sides of the body. An erect, upright posture slightly leaning toward the patient communicates to the patient that the nurse is interested and approachable. This posture combined with intermittent head nodding is a universal sign the listener is acknowledging what is being said by the speaker.[12] A closed stance by the nurse such as crossing arms in front of the chest or placing hands on hips can escalate a patient's stress.[5] Crossed arms can denote insecurity, anger, defensiveness, or anxiety. Speaking to a patient with hands on the hips, especially if the hands are balled into fists, can make the nurse seem aggressive, angry, or territorial.[12] A slumped posture indicates inattention, laziness, or ineptness of the nurse.

Facial expressions are particularly important in therapeutic communication, so nurses should be aware of emotion exhibited through facial expressions and eye contact. It would be appropriate to keep facial expressions neutral or congruent with what is being discussed. The nurse can show compassion, kindness, and interest by exhibiting a small smile, relaxing the muscles of the face, and raising eyebrows slightly.[13] Exaggerated facial expressions can provoke stress and negative reactions in the patient and come across as insincere. Careless expressions of emotion can come across as disgust or judgment, which the patient can misinterpret as directed toward them. In therapeutic communication, the nurse's face and eyes are the primary foci seen by the patient.[11] Eye contact should be direct yet culturally responsive. If eye contact is too excessive for the patient, it can be misconstrued as asserting dominance or influencing. Too little eye contact implies inattention, submission, nervousness, avoidance, or discomfort on the part of the nurse. The use of masks in acute care settings since coronavirus disease has provided an added challenge to meeting the needs of the patient and family causing increased difficulty showing emotion and hearing or understanding what is said.[14] This, too, could cause added stress to the environment and interactions between health-care providers and those entrusted to their care. The traumatic, stressful situation combined with difficulty to understand or see empathy raises the possibility of inappropriate reactivity.

Active listening skills are integral to therapeutic communication and building a strong therapeutic alliance with the patient who has experienced trauma. TIC involves patient-centered and goal-directed communication, so in active listening, the nurse is expected to understand what the patient is saying, respond appropriately, and retain the information.[15] The nurse should look at the patient directly when speaking but also considering the patient's cultural preferences. The nurse should also clear their mind of distracting thoughts including planning out answers. Having a distracted mind may make the nurse miss communication cues or details, which may come across as distracted, unengaged, uncaring, and/or inattentive. As mentioned above, small movements such as nodding signal to the patient that the nurse is paying attention and indicates acceptance and appreciation of what is being said.[12] However, excessive nodding can signal impatience or insincerity. In active listening, the nurse is also providing feedback by reflecting, seeking clarification, restating, and/or paraphrasing. These are types of therapeutic communication techniques that maximize mutual understanding, acknowledge and validate a patient's feelings, and encourage patient autonomy.[15]

Body proxemics is another component of therapeutic communication used within trauma-informed care. Using this technique, the distance between the nurse and patient should be the patient's choice with the ultimate goal being the patient's comfort. Personal space varies with the individual and is separated into 3 zones based on distance: intimate, social, and public spaces. In the United States, research has shown 0 to 4 feet is intimate space and is meant for closer relationships[12]; 4 to 12 feet is social space and is the preferred zone for the nurse to patient relationship in the interview process. When walking, standing, or sitting with the patient, a good rule of thumb is to keep an arm's length away because this distance provides a professional boundary and diminishes any misgivings of unprofessional conduct.[12]

Although an arm's length is recommended, patients should be given permission to change the distance based on their own comfort. Spacing that is too close can be intrusive and threatening while space that is too distant can impair the nurse or patient's ability to see or hear each other. Too much distance can also seem dismissive or impersonal. Remember that sensitivity to this is important to prevent provoking potential traumatic events experienced by this person that the health-care worker may not be aware of. Another recommendation is to meet the patient at the patient's level. This means that if the patient is sitting, the nurse should be sitting at eye level with the patient also. Meeting at the patient's level is important in minimizing power differentials and improving patient satisfaction.[16] Standing over a patient can be perceived as intimidating or hovering. If possible, the patient should also be given a position with a clear eye-line to an exit or a position where they can safely and easily exit if they wish. If the patient is or becomes agitated, this will promote a safe physical space for both patient and nurse.[17]

Haptics, or touch, is an especially important consideration of therapeutic communication with patients who have experienced trauma. The nurse should be careful of communication through touch. Although touch can be therapeutic, the nurse should use their best judgment and always obtain permission from the patient first.[15] If the nurse must touch the patient during an examination, permission from the patient must be granted first or else risk the patient experiencing retraumatization. In patients with trauma, touch can be misinterpreted as threatening, inappropriate, or sexual, so the nurse should be direct and clear about the purpose and necessity of touching.[12]

Another factor that the nurse should maintain awareness of is paralinguistic communication. According to James Borg, a psychological coach and business consultant, "Human communication consists of 93% body language and paralinguistic clues, while only 7% of communication consists of words themselves" (Borg 94–95).[18] Paralinguistic communication is the meaning behind words that are communicated through vocal cues and not necessarily the words being spoken. It is recommended that nurses speak in a softer volume, slower pace, with appropriate intonation that conveys sincerity. The volume, speed, and intonation of the nurse's voice can convey emotion and help a patient relax.[15] Loud volume and fast speech can make a patient feel more anxious and feel hurried. Inappropriate intonation can cause the patient to misinterpret what the nurse is attempting to communicate and create inappropriate reactivity. An example of this is inappropriate intonation that makes the nurse sound sarcastic.

In using trauma-informed care, helping the patient and family to see concern and empathy of the health-care worker can decrease the potential reproduction of trauma-associated reactions and show the sincerity and genuineness of the health-care provider. This is easily done through a patient-centered care mindset and using plain language that the patient can understand. The nurse should practice openness, honesty, and straight-forwardness when communicating with the patient.[15] This enhances the therapeutic alliance by improving trust, transparency, and patient understanding. It also lessens the patient's anxiety.[12] Insincerity can worsen a patient's insecurities or distrust, as well as decrease patient confidence. Disingenuous communication can create misunderstanding, conflict, and missed opportunities to improve patient care.[15] In addition to genuineness, the nurse should use empathy to validate the patient's emotional experience. Empathy promotes welcoming, acceptance, and belief in the patient's situation. Lack of empathy can cause distrust, alienation, and miscommunication.

Culture and society can affect or cause trauma in patients. An example of this is a patient who has experienced racial trauma from discrimination or a hate crime. Cultural humility is an approach to cultural competence and patient-centered care that enhances therapeutic communication. It requires the nurse to constantly self-evaluate their beliefs, be humble, and be willing to adapt to changes. Cultural humility promotes respect and appreciation for the patient as an individual who has lived unique experiences and whose culture has given them meaning and helped shape their reality and identity.[19] One way the nurse can show cultural humility is to ask "about the patient's comfort regarding handshake, eye contact, or personal space."[19] The nurse can also ask the patient about preferred pronouns. For further education on gender, sexuality, and lesbian, gay, bisexual, transgender, queer or questioning (LGBTQ+) identifies, the Safe Zone project can help the nurse provide more inclusive care for patients of differing sexual orientation or gender identity.[19] The nurse should also address the patient's preferred spoken and written language and offer an interpreter if needed. This will help the patient to feel more included and informed in their care. Part of cultural humility is to also self-critique for preconceived opinions and behavior based on stereotypes. Cultivating stereotypes about a patient's culture including religious beliefs, race or ethnicity, and/or gender is close-minded and can breed prejudice in health-care settings.[19] Stereotyping can feel belittling and constraining to the patient.

Finally, silence can be a valuable tool in therapeutic communication if used correctly. Silence should serve a purpose and can signify patience and understanding while awaiting a response from the patient. There is no guidance on how much silence is appropriate but silence should be meaningful, reflective, and contemplative. Too much silence, however, can be awkward or upsetting for the patient and may be perceived as angry or hostile.[15]

Nontherapeutic communication (**Box 3**) should be avoided in order to prevent retraumatization. Nontherapeutic communication can comprise of excessive or intrusive questioning, giving false reassurance, judging, interrupting, and giving advice.[15] When the nurse questions a patient, questioning should be purposeful and consider the patient's state of mind and emotional well-being. Repeating the same questions to a trauma patient can cause retraumatization and discomfort. It feels invasive to the patient and can be overwhelming, stressful, or frustrating.[15] Reassurance can help restore a patient's confidence and hope in times of uncertainty but the nurse should be wary of providing false reassurances that can cause more harm to a trauma patient. False reassurances are not facts, they give false hope, and they make it easy for the patient to blame the nurse if expectations are not met.[15] Active listening and open communication without interruption can engage the patient, promote inclusion, and enhance trust. Interrupting breaks the patient's train of thought, and it shows lack of concern, interest, and caring about what the patient is communicating. Nonjudgmental communication allows patients the ability to be more vulnerable and share more information.

The nonjudgmental nurse is able to be more open-minded and affirms the patient's self-respect. Judgment is perceived as criticism and can cause the patient to feel

---

Box 3
Nontherapeutic communication

Excessive or intrusive questioning
- Avoid repeating the same questions
- Avoid asking questions when the patient is uncomfortable, vulnerable, or closed off

Judging
- Do not criticize the patient or their actions
- Avoid asking "why" questions
- Remove biased and stereotyped words and phrases during communication

Interrupting
- Avoid interrupting the patient when they are speaking

Giving advice
- May be perceived as condescending, judgmental, or dictatorial
- Can become a legal issue
- May be out of the nurse's scope of practice
- May not be evidence-based information

Providing false reassurances
- Could lead to patient disappointment or worsen trauma
- Can lead to the patient blaming the nurse
- Can also become a legal issue

---

stressed or close down communication entirely. Judgment shows the nurse has pre-determined and perhaps biased ideas about the patient and limits the nurse's ability to effectively communicate.[15] TIC aims to improve patient autonomy, and nurses should provide patients with evidence-based patient education. Advice is perceived by the patient as being told what to do and implies lack of trust in the patient's ability to make self-directed decisions. It can also be perceived as condescending, judgmental, and/or dictatorial.

CONSIDERATIONS FOR PRACTICE

The use of TIC should not be confused with trauma-focused psychotherapy modalities. Trauma-specific therapies such as trauma-focused cognitive behavioral therapy, cognitive processing therapy, prolonged exposure therapy, somatic therapies, psychodynamic therapy, and so forth should be performed by health-care professionals who have received specialized training in psychotherapy. Trauma-focused psychotherapies are done in specific settings, whereas TIC can be done in any setting. Although trauma-focused therapies focus on specific traumas and help patients process and cope with these traumas, TIC is a more general approach that aims to not retraumatize the patient while practitioners using TIC should not delve into the patient's traumatic memories or attempt to revive processes impaired by the patient's trauma adaptations. Practitioners using TIC should remember to consider the pervasive presence of trauma and how trauma can affect a patient while trying to improve communication with these patients. Trauma-induced communication is used to better support trauma patients and their health care needs to achieve a more positive health outcome.

Using TIC allows nursing staff to provide respectful and empathetic care to patients who have experienced a traumatic event. It is the foundation for building a therapeutic relationship with the patient and strengthening the therapeutic alliance between nursing and patients. With TIC, there is increased patient buy-in and adherence to treatment plans, which can improve patient outcomes. Conversely, not providing TIC can cause a patient to suffer more stress and distrust health-care providers. Providers could also retraumatize patients through poor communication, which negatively affects care.[20]

The nurse should first understand the prevalence of trauma in the in-patient setting. It is important to be able to recognize signs and symptoms of trauma and recognize patient responses to trauma, which are unique to each patient. The cornerstones of nursing TIC are awareness, sensitivity, and responsiveness.[20] Nurse–patient interactions are constantly adapted to cultivate safety, demonstrate respect, and build trust. Each interaction should begin with an introduction of the nurse's role in the patient's care. There is much self-monitoring done by the nurse when performing TIC.

IMPLICATIONS FOR FUTURE RESEARCH

Little information is found in the literature looking at the impact of trauma-informed care including therapeutic communication in the intensive care setting. In an otherwise stressful and trauma-filled setting, the use of trauma-informed care with special attention focused on the impact of past trauma on the acute traumatic event and trying to minimize the impact those memories might have on acute reactions is instrumental in promoting healthy work environments and healthy collaborative interactions between health-care workers, patients, and families.

Providing insight and education to nurses working in rapidly changing, stress-provoking settings such as the intensive care setting where physical and psychological traumas are prevalent is essential to ensuring effective care for patients and families in the midst of the traumatic event. Further research to determine the relationship between health-care worker training and positive patient/family interaction as well as decreased incidences of escalating interactions being seen is necessary in the orientation and ongoing training of healthcare workers.[11] Cosper and colleagues sought out the management of the perceived lack of empathy in nurses in critical care areas with the use of patient and family advisors.[21] Whether empathy is actual or perceived has yet to be decided but the intervention based on recognizing the need for increased empathy in intensive care nurses was successful in self-reported empathy increasing in participants. Using simulation and discussion with patients and families in a controlled environment, participants were able to explore self-biases and behaviors while gaining input from direct stakeholders in the health-care system.

SUMMARY

Trauma-informed care and communication has a place in every area of nursing care but the impact can especially be felt in the rapidly changing, stressful intensive care unit where the acute traumatic events are prevalent. Recognizing that patients and caregivers have unknown past experiences with trauma and the feelings evoked with these trauma is an important part of providing competent care for individuals and their families. Minimizing inappropriate reactivity in these settings using TIC provides not only a healthy work environment but also an environment where empathetic interactions and communication prevail.

CLINICS CARE POINTS

- Self-awareness of both verbal and nonverbal communication is essential to providing patients experiencing acute trauma a safe environment to be allowed to voice concerns and gain knowledge.

- Health-care workers need to recognize the impact of past, unknown stressors on patient behavior and encourage a therapeutic communication environment to prevent escalation of emotional, confrontational behaviors.
- TIC techniques incorporated into the care of patients can prevent the recurrence of feelings previously experienced in traumatic environments and promote a therapeutic environment.

DECLARATION OF INTERESTS

The authors have nothing to disclose.

REFERENCES

1. Substance abuse and mental health Services Administration (SAMHSHA). "Trauma and violence." Available at: https://www.samhsa.gov/trauma-violence#:~:text=What%20is%20Trauma%20 3F,and%2For%20life%2Dthreatening%20harm. Accessed August 8, 2022.
2. Kaneshiro Neil K. Traumatic events and children. Medline Plus 2020. Available at: https://medlineplus.gov/ency/patientinstructions/000588.htm.
3. Schroeder Krista, et al. A call for trauma-informed intensive care. Nurs Outlook 2021;69(5):717–9. https://doi.org/10.1016/j.outlook.2021.06.001.
4. Brown Taylor, et al. A trauma-informed approach to the medical history: teaching trauma-informed communication skills to first-year medical and dental students. MedEdPORTAL: J Teach Learn Resour 2021;17:11160. https://doi.org/10.15766/mep_2374-8265.11160.
5. Solon Raquelle. How trauma-informed communication improves workplace culture. Available at: https://www.feinet.com/assets/uploads/2020/01/WPQ120_Trauma-Informed-Communication.pdf. Accessed 27 August 2022.
6. Center for Substance Abuse Treatment (US). Trauma-informed care in behavioral health Services. Rockville (MD): substance abuse and mental health Services Administration (US); 2014. (Treatment improvement protocol (TIP) series, No. 57.) chapter 3, understanding the impact of trauma. Available at: https://www.ncbi.nlm.nih.gov/books/NBK207191/.
7. Beattie Jill, et al. Workplace violence perpetrated by clients of health care: a need for safety and trauma-informed care. J Clin Nurs 2019;28:116–24. https://doi.org/10.1111/jocn.14683, 1-2.
8. Hubbard Dena K, et al. Trauma-informed care and ethics consultation in the NICU. Semin Perinatology 2022;46(3). N.PAG. EBSCOhost.
9. Antonacci Rosetta, et al. They can hear the silence: nursing practices on communication with patients. Can J Crit Care Nurs 2018;29(4):36–9. https://www.thefreelibrary.com/They+can+hear+the+silence%3a+Nursing+practices+on+communication+with...-a0640003303.
10. Menschner Christopher, Maul Alexandra. Key ingredients for successful trauma-informed care implementation." Substance Abuse and Mental Health Services Administration. Available at: https://www.samhsa.gov/sites/default/files/programs_campaigns/childrens_mental_health/atc-whitepaper-040616.pdf. Accessed 12 August 2022.
11. Fleishman Joan, et al. Trauma-informed nursing practice. OJIN: The Online J Issues Nurs 2019;24(2). https://doi.org/10.3912/OJIN.Vol24No02Man03. Manuscript 3.

12. Hans Anjali, Hans Emmanuel. Kinesics, haptics and proxemics: Aspects of non –verbal communication. IOSR J Of Humanities And Social Sci 2015;20(2): 47–52. https://www.iosrjournals.org/iosr-jhss/papers/Vol20-issue2/Version4/H02 0244752.pdf.

13. Falconer Caroline J, et al. Compassionate faces: evidence for distinctive facial expressions associated with specific prosocial motivations. PloS one 2019; 14(1). https://doi.org/10.1371/journal.pone.0210283. e0210283.

14. Knollman-Porter Kelly, Burshnic Vanessa L. Optimizing effective communication while wearing a mask during the COVID-19 pandemic. J gerontological Nurs 2020;46(11):7–11. https://doi.org/10.3928/00989134-20201012-02.

15. Halter Margaret. Varcarolis foundations of psychiatric mental health nursing: a clinical approach. 9th ed. Saunders Elsevier; 2022.

16. Swayden Kelli J, et al. Effect of sitting vs. standing on perception of provider time at bedside: a pilot study. Patient Educ Couns 2012;86(2):166–71. https://doi.org/10.1016/j.pec.2011.05.024.

17. Richmond Janet S, et al. Verbal de-escalation of the agitated patient: consensus statement of the American association for emergency psychiatry project BETA de-escalation workgroup. The West J Emerg Med 2012;13(1):17–25. https://doi.org/10.5811/westjem.2011.9.6864.

18. Borg James. Body Language: 7 easy lessons to master the silent language. Pearson Education 2010;94–5.

19. Ranjbar Noshene, et al. Trauma-informed care and cultural humility in the mental health care of people from minoritized communities. Focus (American Psychiatric Publishing) 2020;18(1):8–15. https://doi.org/10.1176/appi.focus.20190027.

20. Brownie Sharon, et al. Therapeutic communication and relationships in chronic and complex care. Nurs Stand (Royal Coll Nurs (Great Britain): 1987) 2016; 31(6):54–63. https://doi.org/10.7748/ns.2016.e9847.

21. Cosper Pam, et al. The impact of patient and family advisors on critical care nurses' empathy. JONA 2018;48(12):622–8. https://doi.org/10.1097/NNA.00000 00000000692.

Moving?

Make sure your subscription moves with you!

To notify us of your new address, find your **Clinics Account Number** (located on your mailing label above your name), and contact customer service at:

Email: journalscustomerservice-usa@elsevier.com

800-654-2452 (subscribers in the U.S. & Canada)
314-447-8871 (subscribers outside of the U.S. & Canada)

Fax number: 314-447-8029

Elsevier Health Sciences Division
Subscription Customer Service
3251 Riverport Lane
Maryland Heights, MO 63043

*To ensure uninterrupted delivery of your subscription, please notify us at least 4 weeks in advance of move.

Printed and bound by CPI Group (UK) Ltd, Croydon, CR0 4YY

03/10/2024

01040466-0012